Quality of Life and Technology Assessment

Monograph of the Council on Health Care Technology

Frederick Mosteller and Jennifer Falotico-Taylor, editors

Institute of Medicine

NATIONAL ACADEMY PRESS
WASHINGTON, D.C. 1989

THE INSTITUTE OF MEDICINE was chartered in 1970 by the National Academy of Sciences to enlist distinguished members of appropriate professions in the examination of policy matters pertaining to the health of the public. In this, the Institute acts under both the Academy's 1863 congressional charter responsibility to be an adviser to the federal government, and its own initiative in identifying issues of medical care, research, and education.

THE COUNCIL ON HEALTH CARE TECHNOLOGY was established in 1986 by the Institute of Medicine of the National Academy of Sciences as a public-private entity to address issues of health care technology and technology assessment. The council is committed to the well-being of patients as the fundamental purpose of technology assessment. In pursuing that goal, the council draws on the services of the nation's experts in medicine, health policy, science, engineering, and industry.

This monograph was supported in part by a grant to the Council on Health Care Technology of the Institute of Medicine from the National Center for Health Services Research and Health Care Technology Assessment of the U.S. Department of Health and Human Services (grant no. HS 0552602). The opinions and conclusions expressed here are those of the authors and do not necessarily represent the views of the Department of Health and Human Services, the National Academy of Sciences, or any of their constituent parts.

Library of Congress Catalog Card Number 89-62585
International Standard Book Number 0-309-04098-1
Additional copies of this report are available from: National Academy Press 2101 Constitution Avenue, NW Washington, DC 20418

S032
Printed in the United States of America
First Printing, October 1989
Second Printing, May 1991

Acknowledgments

This monograph was encouraged by the Council on Health Care Technology as a contribution of the Methods Panel in carrying out its charge to develop and improve the methodologies, techniques, and procedures of technology assessment. Members of the Methods Panel provided comments concerning the original plan and the drafts of this volume. In the early stages William N. Hubbard, Richard A. Rettig, and Enriqueta Bond helped launch the project; Clifford Goodman, Leslie Hardy, and Sharon Baratz have helped it through to completion; Kathleen N. Lohr has participated in the editing.

The council and the Methods Panel greatly appreciate the willingness of the authors to produce their chapters promptly and their help throughout the editing of the monograph.

The staff of the Technology Assessment Group of the Harvard School of Public Health, especially Marie McPherson, and its Sloan Foundation project members have aided in bringing the project to completion. Peg Hewitt contributed to the literature searches. The Health Science Policy Working Group in the Division of Health Policy Research and Education, supported by the Andrew K. Mellon Foundation, has also helped make this monograph possible.

Council on Health Care Technology

Chairman

WILLIAM N. HUBBARD, JR.
Former President, The Upjohn Company

Co-Chairman

JEREMIAH A. BARONDESS
Irene F. and I. Roy Psaty Distinguished Professor of Clinical Medicine, Cornell University Medical College

Members

HERBERT L. ABRAMS
Professor of Radiology, Stanford University School of Medicine

RICHARD E. BEHRMAN
Dean, School of Medicine, Case Western Reserve University

PAUL A. EBERT
Director, American College of Surgeons

PAUL S. ENTMACHER
Senior Vice-President and Chief Medical Director, Metropolitan Life Insurance Company

MELVIN A. GLASSER
Director, Health Security Action Council

BENJAMIN L. HOLMES
Vice-President and General Manager, Medical Products Group, Hewlett-Packard Company

GERALD D. LAUBACH
President, Pfizer Inc.

WALTER B. MAHER
Director, Employee Benefits, Chrysler Corporation

WAYNE R. MOON
Executive Vice-President and Operations Manager, Kaiser Foundation Health Plan, Inc.

LAWRENCE C. MORRIS, JR.
Senior Vice-President, Health Benefits Management, Blue Cross and Blue Shield Association

FREDERICK MOSTELLER
Roger I. Lee Professor (Emeritus), Harvard School of Public Health

MARY O. MUNDINGER
Dean, School of Nursing, Columbia University

ANNE A. SCITOVSKY
Chief, Health Economics Department, Palo Alto Medical Foundation

GAIL L. WARDEN
Chief Executive Officer, Group Health Cooperative of Puget Sound

Methods Panel

Chairman

FREDERICK MOSTELLER
Roger I. Lee Professor (Emeritus), Harvard School of Public Health

Co-Chairman

HERBERT L. ABRAMS
Professor of Radiology, Stanford University School of Medicine

Members

RICHARD E. BEHRMAN
Dean, School of Medicine, Case Western Reserve University

PAUL A. EBERT
Director, American College of Surgeons

DAVID M. EDDY
Center for Health Policy Research and Education, Duke University

JOHN H. FERGUSON
Director, Office of Medical Applications of Research, National Institutes of Health

SUSAN D. HORN
Associate Director, Center for Hospital Finance and Management, Johns Hopkins University School of Hygiene and Public Health

BRYAN R. LUCE
Senior Research Scientist, Battelle Human Affairs Research Centers

ANNE A. SCITOVSKY
Chief, Health Economics Department, Palo Alto Medical Foundation

STEPHEN B. THACKER
Assistant Director for Sciences, Center for Environmental Health, Atlanta, Georgia

ELEANOR TRAVERS
Chair, Task Force on Technology Assessment, Veterans Administration

NORMAN W. WEISSMAN
Director, Division of Extramural Research, National Center for Health Services Research

METHODS PANEL

Preface

In the recent past the interests of different groups concerned with health care have focused on the use of medical technologies—their impacts on safety, efficacy, and effectiveness; cost-effectiveness and cost-benefit; quality; and their social, legal, and ethical implications. The sum of these varied interests is the field of health care technology assessment.

The Council on Health Care Technology was created to promote the development and application of technology assessment in health care and the review of health care technologies for their appropriate use. The council was established as a public-private enterprise at the Institute of Medicine, a component of the National Academy of Sciences, through the Health Promotion and Disease Prevention Amendments of 1984 (P.L. 98-551, later amended by P.L. 99-117). In 1987 the U.S. Congress extended support for the council as a public-private venture for an additional three years (by P.L. 100-177).

The goals and objectives of the council, as stated in the report of its first two years of operation, are "to promote the development and application of technology assessment in medicine and to review medical technologies for their appropriate use. The council is guided in its efforts by the belief that the fundamental purpose of technology assessment is to improve well-being and the quality of care." In pursuing these goals the council seeks to improve the use of medical technology by developing and evaluating the measurement criteria and the methods used for assessment; to promote education and training in assessment methods; and to provide technical assistance in the use of data from published assessments.

The council conducts its activities through several working and liaison panels. Members of these panels reflect a broad set of interested constituencies —physicians and other health professionals, patients and their families, payers for care, biomedical and health services researchers, manufacturers of health-related products, managers and administrators throughout the health care system, and public policymakers. In addition, it carries out councilwide activities that utilize the specific assignments of more than one panel.

This monograph contributes to the series of occasional publications of the council in carrying out its several missions. A guiding principle of the council is a special focus on outcome measures that coincide with patient well-being, quality of health care, and quality of life.

WILLIAM N. HUBBARD, JR., CHAIRMAN
JEREMIAH A. BARONDESS, CO-CHAIRMAN

PREFACE

Contents

1. Conceptual Background and Issues in Quality of Life 1
   Kathleen N. Lohr

2. The Use of Quality-of-Life Measures in Technology Assessment 7
   Jennifer Falotico-Taylor, Mark McClellan, and Frederick Mosteller
   Twelve Applications of Quality-of-Life Measures to Technology Assessment, 14

3. Quality-of-Life Measures in Liver Transplantation 45
   Mark S. Roberts

4. Quality-of-Life Measures and Methods Used to Study Antihypertensive Medications 51
   Sol Levine and Sydney H. Croog

5. The Use of Quality-of-Life Measures in the Private Sector 55
   Bryan R. Luce, Joan M. Weschler, and Carol Underwood

6. Assessing Quality of Life: Measures and Utility 65
   J. Ivan Williams and Sharon Wood-Dauphinee
   Three Sources of Descriptive Information for Quality-of-Life Measures, 83
   Ten Review Forms for Quality-of-Life Measures, 89

7. Applications of Quality-of-Life Measures and Areas for Cooperative Research 116
   Jennifer Falotico-Taylor and Frederick Mosteller

   The Authors 119

CONTENTS

1

Conceptual Background and Issues in Quality of Life

Kathleen N. Lohr

In fields as diverse as health technology assessment, health care quality assurance, and health services research, the hunt for reliable and valid measures of health outcomes intensified greatly in the 1980s. At the same time, the concept of health status expanded to encompass "quality of life." Neither health status nor quality of life is a completely developed concept; neither has behind it a body of literature that fully documents the range or quality of usable measures and instruments. This is demonstrated in the existing literature, which reflects confusion over the appropriate content of these constructs and how they should be measured.

To address some of these gaps in understanding health status and quality of life, the Institute of Medicine's Council on Health Care Technology commissioned this monograph. It selectively surveys the quality-of-life field, offering examples of the use of these types of measures in technology assessment and related applications. Particular attention is given to their use in pharmaceutical trials, where they have received the broadest exposure. Chapter 6 provides basic references for the technical attributes (for example, reliability, validity) of many established measures and also reviews a few less well known measures, especially those used in cancer studies, so that potential users will be able to appreciate their relative advantages and limitations. The final chapter offers some recommendations concerning the appropriate applications of these measures and highlights areas for cooperative research.

CONCEPTUAL BACKGROUND

Potential users of quality-of-life measures need to appreciate the conceptual complexity of this field and the great array of tools available. Misapprehension about what is being measured or poor choices among existing measures can lead users to unfortunate—but avoidable—mistakes. The most important point to understand is that quality of life, health status, functional status, and similar terms are not synonymous; quality of life, in particular, is an inconsistently used concept and is ill-defined in the clinical or health services research literature. Furthermore, the instruments used to assess these variables are not always interchangeable. Finally, the practical inferences one might draw from the application of these measures in clinical or biomedical research, policy research, or even clinical practice could vary dramatically, depending on what one believed one was measuring.

A Continuum of Health-Related Measures

Some experts view these concepts as lying along a health-state continuum: the more restrictive the concept (such as impairment), for instance, the further to the left on the continuum, and the more global the concepts (ultimately including quality of life), the more to the right. Concepts to the right encompass all the domains lying to the left.

Others see these constructs as a set of concentric circles. Dimensions such as functional status are closer to the center and thus are more narrowly defined; quality of life is the largest circle and, again, embodies the broadest set of circumstances or attributes that may affect an individual, including those in the smaller circles.

Health Status

The greatest confusion concerns the distinctions—equivalently, the commonalities—between measures related directly to individual health status and those embracing other attributes of an individual's life.

Health status—sometimes denoted health-related quality of life—itself constitutes a complex, multidimensional construct. A partial list of variables generally recognized in this domain includes survival and life expectancy; various symptom states, such as pain; numerous physiologic states, such as blood pressure or glucose level; physical function states of many sorts, for instance, mobility and ambulation, sensory functioning, sexual functioning, or a range of capacities relating to impairment, disability, and handicap; emotional and cognitive function status, such as anxiety and depression or positive well-being; perceptions about present and future health; and satisfaction with health care (Lohr 1988). Experts generally agree on five distinct health concepts as belonging in the domain of health status—physical health, mental health, social functioning, role functioning, and general health perceptions; some add pain as a sixth key concept (Ware 1987; Mosteller et al. 1989).

Health status measures differ in a number of ways. Some of these constructs (death, pain) are age-old; others (modern notions of functional status, patient satisfaction with care) are quite recent. Some (death, physiologic states) have been defined and can be observed and measured with considerable precision; others (emotional stability, health perceptions) are open to substantial interpretation and are measured with less quantitative rigor. Finally, some can—or must—be measured by someone other than the patient, especially physiologic variables requiring laboratory or other tests; others are assessed only through direct inquiry of a patient or research study subject, primarily through questionnaires.

In the last two decades, numerous health status measures of documented reliability and validity have been developed (McDowell and Newell 1987, Lohr and Ware 1987, Lohr 1989). The Sickness Impact Profile (SIP) (Bergner et al. 1981) is one well-known example of a general health measure. Its 12 dimensions include ambulation, mobility, body care (collectively considered a physical health measure), social interaction, communication, alertness behavior, emotional behavior (collectively, a psychosocial measure), sleep/rest, eating, work, home management, and recreation/pastimes.

In this and similar instruments, the individual is asked to respond to a series of statements about specific components of health; in the case of the SIP, the person is asked to respond "yes" if the statement describes him or her "today" and "is related to your health." Questions concerning activities are phrased in terms of actual performance, not capacity to perform.

In contrast, the General Health Ratings Index was developed as a way to ask people to evaluate their health in general (Davies and Ware 1981). This measure assesses people's views of their own prior, current, and future health and their susceptibility to illness by asking them to respond to questions such as "During the past month, how worried or concerned about your health have you been?" or to label as true or false such state ments as "When there is something going around, I usually catch it." This approach integrates the physical and psychosocial domains tapped more specifically and directly by other health status questionnaires.

Quality-of-Life Measures

A full set of quality-of-life measures would encompass not only the types of measures just mentioned but also a wide range of internal and external attributes of the individual. One expert defines quality of life as "those aspects of life and human function considered essential for living fully" (Mor 1987). (For the most comprehensive review of these measures to date, see the volume of the *Journal of Chronic Diseases* edited by Katz, 1987.) These can include components of one's "environment," such as attributes of housing, neighborhood, or community that relate to comfort, safety, absence of crime, convenience of shopping or commuting to work, and any number of similar material factors. Other environmental aspects of quality of life might involve characteristics of work situations (work load, stressful job relationships).

Other personal or environmental attributes might be included in a comprehensive quality-of-life definition, such as educational attainment or opportunities, income and living standards, and similar financial, social, or demographic elements. Yet others view measures of an individual's ability to cope with short-or long-term stressful situations as an important dimension of quality of life. Notions of coping can then be extended to ideas of the social support network (for example, family, friends, neighbors, co-workers) and of religion and spirituality. One comprehensive listing of quality-of-life variables used in surgical trials, for instance, notes all of the constructs already mentioned (for both health status and quality of life), as well as scales or measures of body image, confidence, self-image, self-esteem, and level of hope (O'Young and McPeek 1987). In sum, concepts of quality of life can be extraordinarily broad, and the interests of clear technology assessment strategy and communication of research results are best served when the health status segment of the continuum is clearly demarcated and appropriate methods and measures are selected.

ISSUES RELATING TO SELECTING HEALTH AND QUALITY-OF-LIFE MEASURES

Questions about the reliability and the face, construct, and convergent/discriminant validity of many of these measures abound, especially for the more diffuse or global quality-of-life instruments. Similar questions can be raised about the feasibility or practicality of administration and about the need or desirability of measuring one or another domain of health or quality of life if (on the grounds of study resources or respondent burden) it means excluding another important, presumably similar domain.

No one answer to these problems can be given. The relevance and value of these measures are determined in large part by the goals of the technology assessments, research studies, or clinical situations in which they may be used. That decided, determining the breadth of measures to be used and selecting the actual measures depends on the quality and suitability of existing instruments for the intended purposes. Most experts concede that no single gold standard exists for assessing all the available measures; they must be evaluated, in part, against each other and in the context of commonly accepted standards of reliability and validity. Most experts also caution, however, against the development of yet new measures, precisely because many good general and specific tools do exist. With respect to the health-related quality-of-life arena, there is growing agreement that the use of one good general health measure, supplemented by diagnosis-or problem-specific instruments, is likely to be the most efficient and rewarding assessment strategy.

For the investigator and clinician interested in this field but lacking the time to review it thoroughly, much can be learned from the successes and failures of past applications of good (or not so good) measures. In addition, information can be amassed about the documented reliability and validity of a number of measures as used for various populations and in health care delivery settings. The remainder of this monograph (and the citations given herein) constitutes a brief overview of the uses, pitfalls, advantages, and limitations of selected health status (health-sensitive quality-of-life) measures, especially in the technology assessment arena. Our aim is to illustrate and describe these measures and the related concepts so that readers can decide whether and when using these measures will improve their research in medical technology assessment.

REFERENCES

Bergner, M., Bobbit, R.A., Carter, W.B., and Gilson, B.S. The Sickness Impact Profile: Development and final revision of a health status measure. Medical Care 19(8):787-805, 1981.

Davies, A.R., and Ware, J.E., Jr. Measuring Health Perceptions in the Health Insurance Experiment. R-2711-HHS. Santa Monica, California, The RAND Corporation, 1981.

Katz, S., ed. The Portugal conference: Measuring quality of life and functional status in clinical and epidemiologic research. Proceedings. Journal of Chronic Diseases 40(6):459-650, 1987.

Lohr, K.N. Outcome measurement: Concepts and questions. Inquiry 25(1):37-50, Spring 1988.

Lohr, K.N., ed. Advances in health status assessment. Proceedings of a conference. Medical Care 27(3):S1-S294 (Supplement), 1989.

Lohr, K.N., and Ware, J.E., Jr., eds. Proceedings of the advances in health assessment conference. Journal of Chronic Diseases 40:S1-S193 (Supplement), 1987.

McDowell, I., and Newell, C. Measuring Health. A Guide to Rating Scales and Questionnaires. New York, Oxford University Press, 1987.

Mor, V. Cancer patients' quality of life over the disease course: Lessons from the real world. Journal of Chronic Diseases 40(6):535-544, 1987.

Mosteller, F., Ware, J.E., Jr., and Levine, S. Finale panel. Comments on the conference on advances in health status assessment. Medical Care 27(3):S282-S294 (Supplement), 1989.

O'Young, J., and McPeek, B. Quality of life variables in surgical trials. Journal of Chronic Diseases 40(6):513-522, 1987.

Ware, J.E., Jr. Standards for validating health measures: Definition and content. Journal of Chronic Diseases 40(6):473-480, 1987.

2

The Use of Quality-of-Life Measures in Technology Assessment

Jennifer Falotico-Taylor, Mark McClellan, and Frederick Mosteller

This chapter contains a set of examples of the application of quality-of-life measures to specific comparative assessments of medical technologies. Rather than representing a comprehensive review of the broad variety of measures described in the literature, these studies illustrate the types of issues likely to arise in efforts to evaluate quality-of-life as a component of technology assessments. Such issues include study design and the limitations and advantages of specific measures, as well as the kinds of information and insights they produce. Quality-of-life indicators have generally been applied to therapies for chronic conditions, for conditions where an increase in length of survival is unlikely, and for conditions with negative consequences of care that may outweigh its benefits. Consequently, the studies may be particularly relevant for clinical trials, drug evaluations, and other analyses to help guide decisions about alternative technologies and treatments in these areas.

LITERATURE REVIEWS

Literature reviews of two successive five-year periods show that the rate of use of quality-of-life measures and the rigor of the methods of study have changed substantially. Najman and Levine (1981) conducted

---

Acknowledgment: We appreciate the advice of J.M. Najman and the editor of *Science and Medicine*, Peter McEwan, in guiding us to James G. Hollandsworth's paper, and we are grateful to Hollandsworth for providing us with a prepublication copy of his paper, thus facilitating our use of the two reviews to indicate the changing situation.

a literature search for uses of quality-of-life measures in technology assessment from 1975 to 1979. They found 23 published studies on the impact of medical care or technology on the quality of life, and only one was a randomized clinical trial. Hollandsworth's 1988 update of this effort found 69 empirically based studies from 1980 to 1984, a threefold increase over the number of papers found by Najman and Levine.

Najman and Levine criticize the "doubtful validity" of the criteria used to measure quality of life in the studies they examined. "Most of the studies (20 out of 23) (87 percent) use only objective indicators" Najman and Levine note, adding, "Researchers appear to have chosen criteria arbitrarily with no regard to the issue of relative priority that might be given to some of the criteria. Nor are the criteria intercorrelated to determine whether, in some instances, there have been systematic and consistent changes in the quality-of-life following medical intervention."

In Hollandsworth's review, 28 out of 69 (41 percent) of the studies used only objective criteria. Almost 60 percent of recent studies have included a subjective measure of quality of life compared with 13 percent in the previous five-year period. Subjective measures require some form of evaluation by the patient. Objective measures include clinical measures, such as survival or the presence of medical complications, as well as other concrete data provided by sources other than the patient. Over half of the studies identified by Hollandsworth used both objective and subjective criteria.

Najman and Levine note that almost all studies in their review concluded that the intervention imposed improved quality of life. Hollandsworth concludes that in the current review approximately half of the studies reported either negative or mixed results. All but one of the seven randomized clinical trials found mixed outcomes or a lack of statistically significant differences between the groups.

Study Design

In the area of study design, some features have improved and others have not. Essentially the same proportion (64 percent) of the studies appearing in the recent five-year period (1980-1984) employed a one-shot case study design with no control-group, as had appeared during the previous five-year period (61 percent). During the same period, however, Hollandsworth found that the proportion of randomized clinical trials had increased from 4 percent to 10 percent.

Approximately 65 percent of the studies reviewed during both five-year periods used samples drawn from "consecutive patients," those patients presenting themselves for treatment, or "all survivors," those patients who have survived for a period of time following treatment. Hollandsworth, however, reports an increase from 2 to 22 in the actual number of studies using matched comparison groups or randomized assignment of subjects to treatment conditions. Sample sizes doubled from an average of 90 to 178 between the first five-year period and the second.

These reviews document that a wide variety of both established and nonestablished quality-of-life measures are currently being used to help give patients a greater voice in appreciating the outcome of medical interventions. The rise in the number of quality-of-life studies reported in the literature suggests that these measures are playing an increasingly important role in both clinical trials and the evaluation of a variety of medical interventions for chronic diseases such as hypertension, coronary disease, renal disease, arthritis, and cancer.

To assist the reader in locating matters of interest in the studies reviewed in this chapter, we have provided several aids. Table 2-1 lists the technologies assessed in each study. At the beginning of each study, we have provided a set of keys describing the technology or treatment assessed, the patient group(s) involved, diagnosis type, measure category, and measure(s) used to assess quality of life. The description of measures or instruments adds information about the kinds of measures available for specific purposes. The comments concluding each summary combine the authors' reflections on their use of quality-of-life measures with our own and stress the value of these measures, along with some caveats to prospective investigators.

The studies reflect a spectrum of approaches and findings; reviewing them collectively can provide a sense of the current scope of assessments of quality of life. In these studies, as well as others we reviewed, we observed a series of recurrent themes. Many researchers encountered some difficulties in the execution and analysis of their studies. In part, limitations emerge from the continuing development of the measures themselves; as their refinement continues, more valid and powerful conclusions should result from their application. In part, however, these limitations also reflect the importance of experimental design in any clinical trial. Such design issues as randomization, double-blinding, standardized implementation, and consideration of patients who withdraw are important whether or not quality-of-life measures are employed.

TABLE 2-1 Technologies Exemplified and Instruments Contributing to the Assessment

Study Number	Technologies Assessed and Instruments Used	Page Number
1	Antihypertensive medications	14
	General Well-Being Adjustment Scale	
	Life Satisfaction Index	
	Physical Symptoms Distress Index	
	Sleep Dysfunction Scale	
	Positive Symptoms Index from the Brief Symptom Inventory	
	Wechsler Memory Scale	
	Reitan Trail-Making Test	
	Social Participation Index	
	Sexual Symptoms Distress Index	
2	Arthritis medications	17
	Health Assessment Questionnaire	
	Keitel Assessment	
	Quality of Well-Being Questionnaire	
	Toronto Activities of Daily Living Questionnaire	
	McGill Pain Questionnaire	
	Pain Ladder Scale	
	10-cm Pain Line	
	Arthritis Categorical Scale	
	Arthritis Ladder Scale	
	Overall Health Ladder Scale, Current	
	Overall Health Ladder Scale, 6-Day Mean	
	RAND Current Health Assessment Measure	
	10-cm Overall Health Scale, by Patient	
	10-cm Overall Health Scale, by Physician	
	Patient Utility Measurement Set	
	Standard Gamble Questionnaire	
	Willingness-to-Pay Questionnaire	
	National Institute of Mental Health (NIMH) Depression Questionnaire	
	RAND General Health Perceptions Questionnaire	
3	Adjuvant chemotherapy	21
	Perceptions of Emotional Distress and Behavioral Disruption	
4	Alternative chemotherapy regimens in advanced breast cancer	23
	Quality of Life Index (QLI)	
	Linear Analogue Self-Assessment (LASA)	

Study Number	Technologies Assessed and Instruments Used	Page Number

5	Counseling for stage IV cancer
	    Cumulative Illness Rating Scale
	    Depression Factor of the Psychiatric Outpatient Mood Scale (POMS)
	    Sherwood's Self-Esteem Scale
	    Cantril's Life Satisfaction Scale
	    Srole's Alienation Scale
	    Rotter's Locus of Control Scale
	    Rapid Disability Rating Scale
		26

6	Surgery for breast cancer
	    NIMH Center for Epidemiologic Studies Depression Scale (CES-D)
	    Body Image Scale (BIS)
		28

7	Cardiac transplant and coronary artery bypass graft surgery
	    Nottingham Health Profile (NHP)
	    Quality of Life Questionnaire
		30

8	Cardiac rehabilitation programs Sickness Impact Profile (SIP)	32

9	Long-term dialysis and renal transplant
	    Quality-of-life indices
	    Physical activity indices
	    Kupfer-Detre System Form 1
	    Kupfer-Detre System Form 2
		34

10	Renal transplantation and dialysis
	    Karnofsky Index
	    Index of Psychological Affect
	    Index of Overall Life Satisfaction
	    Index of Well-Being
	    Work status
		36

11	Case management and usual and customary services for chronically mentally ill patients
	    Social function
	    Affect Balance Scale
	    Self-Esteem Scale
	    Cost-benefit analysis
		39

12	Health insurance payment mechanisms General Health Rating Index	41

NOTE: Page number refers to the page in this chapter where discussion of this application begins.

Not Reinventing the Wheel

Using *established* quality-of-life measures provides special advantages to clinical investigators. This approach frees the investigator from "reinventing the wheel" by employing measures of demonstrated validity, reliability, and relative ease of administration. Moreover, using established measures facilitates the comparison and combination of study results with those obtained by other investigators using the same measures. In this way, larger sample sizes can be accrued by relating similar studies, and a broader range of alternative therapies or patient groups can be compared. For example, given the large number of antihypertensive medications available and the broad variety of patients undergoing therapy, no single experiment can adequately encompass this variety. Comparability of measures makes comparisons across conditions easier, and some established measures make it possible to compare scores with those of the general population. Reliance on established measures can thus promote more effective technology assessments.

At the same time, some studies profitably combine established measures with a limited set of instruments developed by the investigators. This customized approach may be particularly valuable when assessing a technology that involves relatively distinctive quality-of-life features in special populations. In such situations, the investigators can identify the established measures that most closely reflect their experimental interests. They can then supplement these measures with a specific group of items directly reflecting their concerns. For example, elderly patients or individuals from different socioeconomic or cultural backgrounds may require particular modifications in the content or administration of some indicators. Similarly, assessments of alternative surgical procedures for breast cancer require special emphasis on body image and sexual function.

THE VALUE OF ASSESSING QUALITY OF LIFE AS AN OUTCOME

Measures of quality of life promote an emphasis on issues of direct importance to patients that are only indirectly reflected in clinical measures and interpersonal communication. Consequently, they complement the more traditional sources of information for evaluating therapies and choosing appropriate treatments. For example, quality-of-life indicators can provide reliable and valid data on the side effects of drugs and on iatrogenic consequences of procedures. Such data help to distinguish between alternative treatments that are equivalent in clinical and other objective measures.

Combining quality-of-life measures with clinical indicators and other objective outcome data produces a more comprehensive picture of the technology being assessed. This combination may promote a more sophisticated analysis of technologies than either approach alone might permit. For example, studies involving combinations of measures for end-stage renal disease patients not only provided more information on the relative advantages of renal transplants, but also indicated that objective and subjective clinical measures correlated poorly in all experimental groups—that is, the patients' subjective experience of disease correlated poorly with their clinical status.

Work Status

Work status as a measure of quality of life requires special comment. Work status before and following treatment has major interest for society and for patients. Work status depends on whether or not patients were employed at the time of their treatment, their age, how patients view their work both before and after treatment, the support after treatment, and the outcome of treatment. We are told by experts that some patients put off important operations because they fear being discharged from their positions after treatment. Others are eager to have the treatment, regardless of the consequences. Because the latter may receive disability payments or other financial support, they may be able to sustain themselves without returning to work or with partial work, especially if they do not find their work gratifying. Social policies in various countries and social units offer differing degrees of support to those who retire or are disabled at various ages, making situations less comparable. Thus, work status, although it has important social and economic consequences, has several variables muddying its resolution; therefore it cannot, without deeper investigation, be regarded as a very direct measure of the success of therapy or the quality of life of the patient. Some patients will find their quality of life reduced if their work is no longer available to them, and others will be very satisfied.

DIAGNOSIS—AN OPEN PROBLEM

None of the studies given in this chapter deals with the improved quality of life that accompanies the reduction of uncertainty about the disease state of the patient. Measuring the benefit of such anxiety reduc tion may be difficult, and no established measures are available. Herbert L. Abrams, co-chairman of the Methods Panel of the Institute of Medicine Council on Health Care Technology, emphasizes that a large proportion of patient visits to physicians deal with complaints for which no therapy is available. The complaints themselves may bear heavily on the quality of the patients' lives. Information alone may appropriately allay the anxiety of the patients and thus improve their quality of life.

In some areas, diagnosis can be made with a high degree of accuracy, and appropriate patient management can be undertaken if disease is present or reassurance may be given if it is not. Signs and symptoms of brain tumors, gastrointestinal distress, and impending coronary problems produce anxiety that can often be reduced by diagnosis and education. Even when the news is bad, the resolution of uncertainty and starting an active management plan may improve the patients' quality of life.

ROLES OF THE EXAMPLES

Finally, these studies collectively indicate that quality-of-life measurements can have a significant impact on the conclusions in clinical technology assessments. They can help differentiate among chemotherapy regimens, antihypertensive medications, and many other technologies that appear similar according to other criteria. They can demonstrate the value of some therapies that do not prolong life for terminally ill patients, and they can help gauge the effectiveness of treatment when no alternative exists. They can help target the concern of health providers to those areas where patients think their lives are most affected, thereby contributing to the therapeutic process. For all of these reasons, quality-of-life measures enable the assessment of an important additional dimension in the evaluation of health care interventions.

TWELVE APPLICATIONS OF QUALITY-OF-LIFE MEASURES TO TECHNOLOGY ASSESSMENT

Study 1. Antihypertensive Medications

Croog, S.H., Levine, S., Testa, M.A., Brown, B., Bulpitt, C.J., Jenkins, C.D., Klerman, G.L., and Williams, G.H. The effects of antihypertensive therapy on the quality of life. New England Journal of Medicine 314(26):1657-1664, 1986.

THE USE OF QUALITY-OF-LIFE MEASURES IN TECHNOLOGY ASSESSMENT

Key

Technology Assessed: Relative effects of captopril, methyldopa, and propranolol
Patient Group: Adults
Diagnosis Type: Essential hypertension
Measure Category: Physical, psychological, and social
Measures: General Well-Being Adjustment Scale, Life Satisfaction Index, Physical Symptoms Distress Index, Sleep Dysfunction Scale, Positive Symptoms Index from the Brief Symptom Inventory, Wechsler Memory Scale, Reitan Trail-Making Test, Social Participation Index, Sexual Symptoms Distress Index

Description of Measures

General Well-Being Adjustment Scale. This scale consists of six subscales: anxiety, depression, general health, positive well-being, self-control, and vitality.

Life Satisfaction Index. This index assesses satisfaction in fourteen areas including marriage, finances, standard of living, housing, and degree of social participation.

Physical Symptoms Distress Index. This index evaluates the degree of distress from symptoms such as lethargy, dry mouth, loss of sense of taste, nightmares, and feeling faint or light-headed.

Sleep Dysfunction Scale. This scale measures the frequency of problems in falling or remaining asleep, early awakening, or awakening tired.

Positive Symptom Index from the Brief Symptom Inventory. This index measures the degree of depression, anxiety, hostility, somatization, and obsessive-compulsiveness.

Wechsler Memory Scale. This scale assesses neuropsychological function based on one's ability to reproduce diagram images.

Reitan Trail-Making Test. This test assesses visuo-motor speed and coordination.

Social Participation Index. This index assesses the degree of participation in social events.

Sexual Symptoms Distress Index. This index assesses distress in areas such as sexual desire or impotence.

Purpose of the Study

Croog et al. compared the effects of captopril, methyldopa, and propranolol on the quality of life of men with mild to moderate essential hypertension.

Methods

Using a randomized double-blind clinical trial, Croog et al. assessed the impact of captopril, methyldopa, and propranolol on the quality of life of 626 white men, aged 21 to 65, with a diagnosis of mild to moderate essential hypertension. They used several quality-of-life measures described above. A placebo was administered to all subjects for a one-month period. This was followed by a six-month active treatment phase, during which patients were randomly assigned to receive one of the three medications. Both the patients and investigators were blinded as to study assignment. Interviews were carried out at the beginning of the study, and again at one-, three-, and six-month intervals.

Results and Conclusions

In the captopril group, 8 percent of patients withdrew following adverse reactions, as did 20 percent of patients in the methyldopa group and 13 percent of patients in the propranolol group. Patients treated with captopril reported a statistically significant six-month improvement in general well-being, work performance, cognitive functioning, and life satisfaction. Patients treated with methyldopa improved only in the area of cognitive functioning, and they worsened in the areas of depression, work performance, sexual functioning, physical symptoms, and life satisfaction. Patients treated with propranolol reported improved cognitive functioning and social participation, but they reported more sexual dysfunction and physical symptoms. Compared with patients receiving captopril, 20 percent more patients treated with methyldopa and 15 percent more patients treated with propranolol reported a worsening in general well-being.

Croog et al. note a close association between withdrawal from therapy because of adverse reactions and the drug's effect on quality of life. They suggest that withdrawal may be an index of noncompliance, a serious problem for physicians treating hypertension because many patients perceive the side effects of the drugs to be more troubling than their "seem ingly symptomless disease." The short-term withdrawal rates in this six-month study may actually underestimate the potential long-term noncompliance rates for patients on antihypertensive medications.

Comments

The generalizability of this study is limited by the study population. For example, the results may not apply to other hypertensive groups, such as women, the elderly, lower-income persons, and different ethnic groups.

The study demonstrates that quality-of-life measures highlight the iatrogenic effects of drugs that successfully control blood pressure, but with differential effects on various aspects of the physical state, emotional well-being, sexual and social functioning, and cognitive ability of patients.

The study is also important because it uses several measurement instruments to reinforce its conclusions, and because it is a major quality-of-life-oriented clinical trial funded by a pharmaceutical company, thus indicating the potential role for quality-of-life considerations in both clinical decisionmaking and marketing.

Study 2. Arthritis Medications

Bombardier, C., Ware, J., Russell, I.J., Larson, M., Chalmers, A., and Read, J.L. Auranofin therapy and quality of life in patients with rheumatoid arthritis. Results of a multicenter trial. The American Journal of Medicine 81(4):565-578, 1986.

Key

Technology Assessed: Auranofin therapy
Patient Group: Adults
Diagnosis Type: Rheumatoid arthritis
Measure Category: Clinical, psychological, functional performance, pain, global impression, and utility
Measures: Health Assessment Questionnaire; Keitel Assessment; Quality of Well-Being Questionnaire; Toronto Activities of Daily Living Questionnaire; McGill Pain Questionnaire; Pain Ladder Scale; 10-cm Pain Line; Arthritis Categorical Scale; Arthritis Ladder Scale; Overall Health Ladder Scale, Current; Overall Health Ladder Scale, 6-Day Mean; RAND Current Health Assessment Measure; 10-cm Overall Health Scale,

by Patient; 10-cm Overall Health Scale, by Physician; Patient Utility Measurement Set; Standard Gamble Questionnaire; Willingness-to-Pay Questionnaire; National Institute of Mental Health Depression Questionnaire; RAND General Health Perceptions Questionnaire

Description of Measures

Health Assessment Questionnaire (HAQ). The HAQ specifies eight areas of daily function, each with two to three activities. The patient scores the degree of difficulty in performing the activities on a scale from 3 (unable) to 0 (without difficulty).

Keitel Assessment. This measure requires patients to assess their degree of difficulty in performing each of 23 range-of-motion tasks. Scores range from 98 (worst) to 0.

Quality of Well-Being Questionnaire (QWB). The QWB is used to assess the functional limitations of patients caused by their health within the previous six days in the areas of mobility, physical activity, and social activity.

Toronto Activities of Daily Living Questionnaire. This questionnaire is used to determine how much performance has changed over the course of the study in 21 areas of daily living. Response scores range from -4 (worst) to 1.

McGill Pain Questionnaire. This questionnaire consists of 20 groups of words from which patients select those that describe their current pain status. Response scores range from 0 (worst) to 6.

Pain Ladder Scale. This scale was designed for this study. It represents 10 degrees of pain from "none" to "severe." Using the patient's degree of pain experienced for each of the past six days, investigators calculate a mean score.

10-Centimeter Pain Line. This measure uses a visual analogue, noncalibrated line anchored by the terms "excruciating" and "none." The patients mark a spot on the line to indicate their degree of pain.

Arthritis Categorical Scale. This scale asks patients to describe their current arthritic symptoms by selecting one of five responses ranging from "very poor" to "very good."

Arthritis Ladder Scale. This scale is used to measure 10 degrees of difficulty associated with arthritis from "most severe problems" to "no problems." The patient records the degree of difficulty experienced for each of the past six days, and this record produces the patient's mean score.

Overall Health Ladder Scale, Current. This scale represents 10 degrees of health ranging from "least desirable" to "most desirable." Patients select the degree of overall health corresponding to their current health status.

Overall Health Ladder Scale, 6-Day Mean. This scale averages the responses to overall health for each of the past six days.

RAND Current Health Assessment Measure. This measure consists of 19 statements about current health that patients classify from "definitely true" to "definitely false." Responses range from a score of 9 (worst) to 45.

10-Centimeter Overall Health Scale, by Patient. This self-assessment scale uses a visual analogue technique. The noncalibrated line is anchored by the terms "poor" and "perfect" to describe overall health. Scores range from 0 (worst) to 10.

10-Centimeter Overall Health Scale, by Physician. This scale is similar to the previous scale, except that the physician indicates the health status of the patient.

Patient Utility Measurement Set (PUMS). The PUMS measures the patients' perceptions of their current health state relative to their recollected health state at the beginning of the study and to a state of complete health.

Standard Gamble Questionnaire. This questionnaire, developed for this study, asks patients to choose between their current health state and a hypothetical treatment with systematically varied chances of complete recovery or death. A higher risk indicates a worse condition.

Willingness-to-Pay Questionnaire. This questionnaire was also developed for this study. It asks patients to report the percentage of income they would pay for a hypothetical arthritis cure. A higher percentage indicates a worse condition.

National Institute of Mental Health Depression Questionnaire. This questionnaire asks patients to report how many of 20 depressive thoughts or attitudes they experienced within the last seven days. Scores range from 60 (worst) to 0.

RAND General Health Perceptions Questionnaire. This questionnaire has 36 true or false statements reflecting patients' attitudes toward past and future health care and outlook. Responses are combined to produce an overall score ranging from 0 (worst) to 110.

Purpose of the Study

Bombardier et al. assessed the effect of auranofin in patients with rheumatoid arthritis.

Methods

Bombardier et al. conducted a six-month, randomized double-blind study to assess the quality of life of 154 patients, aged 18 to 65 years, who received auranofin in the treatment of rheumatoid arthritis and 149 patients who received a placebo. They grouped clinical and quality-of-life measures into four composites — clinical, functional, global, and pain — to minimize the problems associated with multiple comparisons. Patients completed clinical and quality-of-life measures two weeks before medication was given and on the day it was first administered. Investigators used score means as baseline values and reassessed these means at six months. They assessed utility at the fifth month of treatment.

Results and Conclusions

The investigators found no significant differences between treatment groups in any of the four composites at baseline. At the six-month comparison, the auranofin group had significantly greater improvement than did the placebo group in the clinical, functional, and global impression dimensions. Though not statistically significant, the auranofin group also showed more improvement in the pain composite than did the placebo group.

More patients in the auranofin group withdrew, because of adverse side effects such as diarrhea and abdominal pain, than did patients in the placebo group. These side effects, however, did not persist after discontinuation of therapy. Most adverse episodes were "mild or transient," and the majority of patients remained in the study.

Comments

Bombardier et al. offer some caveats to prospective investigators with respect to choosing from among several general and arthritis-specific questionnaires. They note that within the functional composite, the Quality of Well-Being Scale, the Keitel Assessment instrument, and the Health Assessment Questionnaire showed "comparable sensitivity to treatment despite distinct differences in their content, detail, length, mode of administration, and method of scoring." The best choice appears to be the HAQ, because it is the simplest and shortest self-administered questionnaire. Within the pain composite, the McGill Pain Questionnaire, Pain Ladder Scale, and 10-Centimeter Pain Line were also comparably sensitive to treatment. The most efficient index appears to be the brief, well-established, 10-Centimeter Pain Line (visual analogue scale).

The investigators found an inconsistent pattern of sensitivity among measures of global impression; the self-administered, five-point Arthritis Categorical Scale demonstrated a highly significant treatment effect that was consistent with the other composite measures.

Of the three utility measures, the PUMS was more sensitive to treatment effect than the Standard Gamble or Willingness-to-Pay Questionnaire. Neither the National Institute of Mental Health (NIMH) Depression Questionnaire nor the RAND General Health Perceptions Questionnaire recorded a significant difference between the two groups.

The use of over 20 "nontraditional" measures, in addition to five standard clinical measures, highlights the availability of several general or arthritis-specific quality-of-life indices. This simultaneous appraisal of many measures can help clinical investigators to identify and select the most sensitive indices of quality of life for their patients. The study demonstrates a method for introducing and assessing newly developed indices. It also provides an opportunity for other researchers to select from among the more than 20 measures used in this investigation for their own research purposes.

Study 3. Adjuvant Chemotherapy

Meyerowitz, B.E., Sparks, F.C., and Spears, I.K. Adjuvant chemotherapy for breast carcinoma. Cancer 43(5):1613-1618, 1979.

Key

Technology Assessed: Adjuvant chemotherapy
Patient Group: Adult women
Diagnosis Type: Breast carcinoma
Measure Category: Psychological, physical, and social function
Measures: Perceptions of Emotional Distress and Behavioral Disruption

Description of Measures

Patients rated their perceptions of emotional distress and behavioral disruption in five areas: marital/family relationships, sexual relationships, financial situation, general level of activity, and level of work-related activity. Patients responded to each area on a seven-point scale ranging from "very positive" to "very negative"; the midpoint of the scale represented no change from pretreatment quality of life. They responded to the question "Would you recommend [this therapy] to [your] best friend if she were in the same situation?" on a five-point scale, ranging from the recommendation that she definitely be involved to the recommendation that she definitely not be involved in the adjuvant program.

Purpose of the Study

Meyerowitz et al. assessed the effect of adjuvant chemotherapy for stage II breast carcinoma on the quality of life of postmastectomy patients.

Methods

The investigators selected 50 consecutive, postmastectomy patients, by order of their appointments, from among those patients actively participating in the University of California at Los Angeles (UCLA) Breast Cancer Adjuvant Program. These patients had no evidence of metastases, were free of other major illnesses, and consented to participate in the study. A psychologist, using a structured interview format, asked the women about their perceptions of emotional distress and behavioral disruption in the areas of marital/family relationships, sexual relationships, financial situation, general level of activity, and level of work-related activity. The psychologist also asked whether the women would recommend participation in the program to their best friend.

Results and Conclusions

All interviewed women reported that participation in the adjuvant treatment program had resulted in adverse behavioral and emotional changes in their lives. In the area of marital/family relationships, 23 percent of the women reported increased disruption. In the area of sexual relationships, 17 percent reported marked decreases in sexual activity;

none of the women reported improved sexual experience. Approximately half of the women attributed increased financial burden to lost income and increased medical expenses. The women reported a decrease in both general and work-related levels of activity as the most frequent and marked effect of adjuvant chemotherapy. Additionally, 45 percent of the women reported that their job status had been adversely affected since they had begun chemotherapy.

This distress and disruption was more severe during the second treatment period than during the first or third periods. Nearly all of the women reported adverse physical side effects, such as fatigue, nausea, nervousness, and irritability. These side effects were not, however, significantly related to the reported level of distress and disruption.

Sixty percent of the women reported that they believed their anxiety and fear were reduced through the adjuvant treatment program. Despite the adverse effects, 74 percent claimed they would recommend participation in a similar program to a friend.

Comments

The use of quality-of-life measures in the treatment of stage II breast carcinoma informs investigators of the areas where distress and disruption usually occur. This knowledge may enable medical staff to improve preparation of patients for adjuvant chemotherapy and may help patients by letting them know that their reactions are similar to those of other women. Further, Meyerowitz et al. concluded that the physical side effects of treatment do not account for all of the stress experienced by these women. Thus, the use of quality-of-life measures shows that a "discussion of only the possible physical effects would not prepare a patient fully for adjuvant chemotherapy."

Study 4. Alternative Chemotherapy Regimens in Advanced Breast Cancer

Coates, A., Gebski, V., Bishop, J.F., Jeal, P.N., Woods, R.L., Snyder, R., Tattersall, M.H., Byrne, M., Harvey, V., and Gill, G. Improving the quality of life during chemotherapy for advanced breast cancer. A comparison of intermittent and continuous treatment strategies. New England Journal of Medicine 317 (24):1490-1495, 1987.

Key

Technologies Assessed: Intermittent versus continuous palliative chemotherapy (doxorubicin/cyclophosphamide [DC] or cyclophosphamide/methotrexate/fluorouracil/prednisone [CMFP])
Patient Group: Patients undergoing chemotherapy
Diagnosis Type: Advanced (metastatic) breast cancer
Measure Category: Global well-being, physical status, and mood or affect
Measures: Quality of Life Index (QLI), Linear Analogue Self-Assessment (LASA)

Description of Measures

Quality of Life Index. This index, completed by each patient and her physician, consists of five sections dealing with the areas of work, finances, symptoms, life-style, and expectations.
Linear Analogue Self-Assessment. This is a self-administered measure of physical well-being, mood, pain, nausea and vomiting, and appetite. Investigators derived a uniscale from these measures, summarizing overall quality of life.

Purpose of the Study

Alternative therapies for patients with advanced cancer are not expected to produce substantial differences in clinical outcomes. For this reason, the investigators sought to supplement their evaluation of treatments (DC versus CMFP, intermittent versus continuous) with an assessment of patients' quality of life.

Methods

Coates et al. randomized 308 patients, enrolled at 13 institutions in Australia and New Zealand between June 1982 and June 1985, to receive either intermittent or continuous regimens of DC or CMFP, based on progression of disease. Investigators stratified these patients by institution, clinical performance status, and previous treatment with adjuvant chemotherapy. The researchers based their comparisons of scores on quality-of-life measures on changes in the scores of each patient during treatment. Patients thus served as their "own controls."

Using linear regression, the investigators compared the effects of continuous versus intermittent treatment, the combination of chemotherapeutic agents, and any interaction between these variables. In addition to using quality-of-life measures, the investigators evaluated the patients clinically for indications of the effectiveness of treatment.

Results and Conclusions

Coates et al. excluded all patients at one institution from the analyses because many of their surveys were not completed. They analyzed scores from the remaining patients in two sets. The first set consisted of self-assessments by 133 patients (68 percent of the original group) and physician assessments of 149 patients (76 percent of the original group), for whom baseline scores and scores after completion of three cycles of chemotherapy were available. Investigators noted no significant differences between the groups during this phase.

The second set of data included patients who remained in the study after the two treatment approaches diverged. These data were based on the 83 patients (68 percent) who completed the LASA forms and the 98 patients (78 percent) for whom physicians completed quality-of-life assessments. The investigators noted that the patients for whom quality-of-life data were unavailable did not differ from the others in the clinical measures of response to treatment, survival, or toxic side effects. The investigators calculated single average values, using all the available forms for each patient, and compared these scores with the three-cycle baseline scores. They found that every quality-of-life endpoint was significantly better in the continuous therapy group.

Intermittent therapy was associated with significantly worse clinical results. Response to treatment was poorer, time to disease progression was shorter, and survival time was shorter. Except for nausea and vomiting, no significant differences between the two chemotherapeutic combinations were observed, either in clinical or quality-of-life measures.

Comments

This study compared palliative treatments for survival and disease progression, as well as patients' quality of life. Results demonstrate that intermittent therapy is inferior in palliative treatment for patients with advanced breast cancer in both clinical and quality-of-life measures. This suggests that improved quality of life for patients with advanced breast cancer is associated with clinical response of the tumors to treatment. These results may not be generalizable to therapy at an earlier stage of the disease, or to other types of intermittent treatment.

The quality-of-life measures used in this study demonstrate the effectiveness of palliative chemotherapy in improving the quality of life of terminally ill cancer patients. Similar investigations may be possible for other types of metastatic cancer where the probability of survival is low, and where it is unclear whether chemotherapy toxicity is outweighed by a low probability that tumor response will lead to symptom relief.

Study 5. Counseling for Stage IV Cancer

Linn, M.W., Linn, B.S., and Harris, R. Effects of counseling for late stage cancer patients. Cancer 49(5):1048-1055, 1982.

Key

Technology Assessed: Counseling for stage IV cancer
Patient Group: Adult men with incurable cancer
Diagnosis Type: Stage IV cancer
Measure Category: Psychological function
Measures: Cumulative Illness Rating Scale, Depression Factor of the Psychiatric Outpatient Mood Scale (POMS), Sherwood's Self-Esteem Scale, Cantril's Life Satisfaction Scale, Srole's Alienation Scale, Rotter's Locus of Control Scale, Rapid Disability Rating Scale

Description of Measures

Cumulative Illness Rating Scale. This scale assesses the degree of impairment to 13 body systems on five-point scales.

Depression Factor of the POMS. This measure asks patients to rate adjectives such as "blue" or "sad" on a four-point scale from "not at all" to "extremely" to describe their predominant mood over the past week.

Sherwood's Self-Esteem Scale. This scale asks patients to choose between 14 bipolar adjectives, such as "useful-useless" to describe their present level of self-esteem.

Cantril's Life Satisfaction Scale. This 9-item scale with an 11-rung ladder measures life satisfaction.

Srole's Alienation Scale. This 9-item scale uses an agree/disagree format for statements that measure alienation.

Rotter's Locus of Control Scale. This scale asks patients to choose between pairs of statements to measure how much they perceive themselves to be externally controlled or personally controlled.

Rapid Disability Rating Scale. This 16-item scale assesses functional status at baseline and follow-up.

Purpose of the Study

Linn et al. assessed the impact of psychosocial counseling on quality of life, functional status, and survival in end-stage cancer patients. The investigators tested three hypotheses: (1) that counseling improves quality of life by decreasing depression and alienation and increasing life satisfaction, self-esteem, and internal control; (2) that if quality of life is enhanced, functional status will be higher in experimental patients because the course of illness is influenced by emotional state; and (3) that if patients feel better about themselves and function at a higher level physically, their length of survival might be extended.

Methods

Linn et al. randomly assigned 120 end-stage cancer patients between the ages of 45 and 77 to two groups. These patients were judged to have between 3 and 12 months of survival remaining, were alert and communicative, and gave informed consent to join an experimental ($n = 62$) or control ($n = 58$) group. The investigators assessed the patients' quality of life and functional status before random assignment by a predetermined sealed envelope method and at 1, 3, 6, 9, and 12 months, for as long as patients survived. Nurses, blinded to the patients' treatment assignment, collected the data. A physician completed the Cumulative Illness Rating Scale. The investigators compared groups for baseline differences and at follow-up for survivors.

Results and Conclusions

The investigators found no significant differences between the groups in cancer type, treatment, and degree of impairment initially and at the one-month follow-up. At all subsequent follow-ups, experimental patients showed more positive changes than control patients. At the three-month follow-up, their depression was significantly decreased. Over time, both life satisfaction and self-esteem were significantly increased for the experimental patients.

The experimental group reported less alienation and perceived more internal control. The investigators report that "in all instances, quality-of-life variables showed significant change in favor of the experimental patients . . . with those living the full 12 months showing the most significant gains." Other variables, such as number of days in the hospital during each follow-up time, number of readmissions, degree of compliance with the medical regimens, number of complications, additional illnesses diagnosed, and changes in treatment plan did not differ significantly between groups.

These findings support the investigators' first hypothesis, that counseling improves quality of life. Their theory that changes in quality of life would be accompanied by significant changes in physical functioning was not proved. The patients with improved quality of life did not have increased quantity of life. The investigators state that the goal of therapy was not to extend life but rather to enrich it. They theorize that perhaps intervention at an earlier stage of illness could significantly influence survival.

Comments

The investigators note several problems in this study. Therapy was carried out by only one individual. Only patients who could communicate verbally were seen, and those who met the study criteria never progressed to stages where they could not be interviewed.

As this study demonstrates, quality of life need not correlate with functional status. Quality-of-life measurements can offer information about the interaction between psychological and physical dimensions of functioning and may offer guidance in counseling dying patients and their families.

Study 6. Surgery for Breast Cancer

Lasry, J.C., Margolese, R.G., Poisson, R., Shibata, H., Fleischer, D., Lafleur, D., Legault, S., and Taillefer, S. Depression and body image following mastectomy and lumpectomy. Journal of Chronic Diseases 40(6):529-534, 1987.

Key

Technology Assessed: Alternative surgical therapies for curable breast cancer—total mastectomy, lumpectomy, and lumpectomy plus auxiliary irradiation (all groups also received chemotherapy for lymph node metastases)
Patient Group: Women with potentially curable breast cancer
Diagnosis Type: Breast cancer
Measure Category: Psychological and physical
Measures: National Institute of Mental Health (NIMH) Center for Epidemiologic Studies Depression Scale (CES-D), Body Image Scale (BIS)

Description of Measures

NIMH Center for Epidemiologic Studies Depression Scale. This 20-item scale measures symptoms of depression in the general population. It has two subscales: Positive Affect, consisting of 4 items based on the presence or absence of specific affective states, and Depressive Symptoms, consisting of 16 items based on pathognomonic responses related to psychiatric symptoms. Higher scores reflect the presence of more symptoms.

Body Image Scale (BIS). This seven-item scale was adapted by the investigators from an instrument developed by Steinberg et al. (1985). Patients rate their perceptions of physical attractiveness, femininity, breast appearance, and sexual attractiveness.

Patients rated their fear of recurrence and perceptions of their families' fears on a scale from 1 to 4.

Purpose of the Study

Lasry et al. assessed quality-of-life differences in depression and body image between alternative surgical and radiation therapies for patients with potentially curable breast cancer.

Methods

The investigators studied 123 Montreal patients with potentially curable breast cancer, matched for various socioeconomic variables, in the B-06 National Surgical Adjuvant Breast Project.

Results and Conclusions

The global depression score in all breast cancer patient groups was about twice that of the healthy adult population, but no significant differences in this global score among the patient groups were observed. The lumpectomy/radiotherapy subgroup had significantly higher CES-D scores. Patients undergoing total mastectomy had significantly lower BIS scores than lumpectomy patients on six of the seven items, while the two lumpectomy groups had scores similar to each other. No significant differences existed among the groups in ratings of fear of recurrence.

Comments

Lasry et al. noted that although the therapeutic methods were comparable in clinical effectiveness, some differences were revealed by the quality-of-life measures. They attribute the higher depressive symptom scores in the lumpectomy/radiotherapy group to greater depression and anxiety associated with radiotherapy. They noted that radiotherapy does not seem to influence body image. In reviewing recent work concerning the psychosocial consequences of breast surgery, they categorize research into three main areas: psychological distress (feelings and emotions aroused by cancer), daily life impact (physical discomfort, impact on body image, reduction in activity, sleep disturbance, sexual difficulties), and fears (of cancer itself, its recurrence, death, disfigurement, loss of femininity). They note that their study indicates a higher prevalence of depression in breast cancer patients than in the general population regardless of treatment, and that there is a significantly better personal body image associated with lumpectomy.

Study 7. Cardiac Transplant and Coronary Artery Bypass Graft Surgery

Wallwork, J., and Caine, N. A comparison of the quality of life of cardiac transplant patients and coronary artery bypass graft patients before and after surgery. Quality of Life and Cardiovascular Care 1(7)September/October:317-331, 1985.

THE USE OF QUALITY-OF-LIFE MEASURES IN TECHNOLOGY ASSESSMENT

Key

Technologies Assessed: Cardiac transplant and coronary artery bypass graft surgery
Patient Group: Adults
Diagnosis Type: Coronary disease
Measure Category: Psychological, physical, and social function
Measures: Nottingham Health Profile (NHP), Quality of Life Questionnaire

Description of Measures

Nottingham Health Profile (NHP). The NHP comprises two parts. Part I consists of a set of 38 yes or no statements relating to six dimensions of social functioning: physical mobility, pain, sleep, energy, social isolation, and emotional reaction. Part II lists seven yes or no statements that refer to the effects of health problems on occupation, ability to perform tasks at home, social life, relationships, sexual functioning, hobbies and interests, and holidays.

Quality of Life Questionnaire. This questionnaire has five sections: profession, financial aspects, assessment of symptoms, general life-style, and expectations. There are 30 questions in all, most requiring a yes or no response.

Purpose of the Study

Wallwork and Caine compared the quality of life of cardiac transplant patients with those of coronary artery bypass graft (CABG) patients.

Methods

Wallwork and Caine compared the NHP scores of two groups. The first included 84 pre-CABG patients, 64 CABG patients three months after surgery, and 32 CABG patients one year after surgery. The second group included 61 pretransplant patients, 30 patients three months after transplant, and 24 patients one year after transplant. CABG and transplant procedures were performed in the United Kingdom. Although transplant patients received the NHP and Quality of Life Questionnaire preoperatively and at the three-month and one-year intervals, the investi gators had just begun to administer the Quality of Life Questionnaire to the CABG group at the time of publication.

Results and Conclusions

Part I of the NHP revealed that presurgical transplant patients were significantly less healthy than presurgical CABG patients in the areas of physical mobility, sleep, and energy; they were also more socially isolated. This is probably because all potential transplant patients have end-stage cardiac disease and experience significantly more restrictions and functional problems than CABG patients. Nevertheless, at the one-year follow-up, the only difference between the groups was in the area of energy: the transplant patients reported more energy than the CABG patients. For transplant patients, the area of life that reflected the greatest improvement on Part II of the NHP was the ability to perform tasks in the home. Although CABG patients reported a similarly high rate of improvement in this area, they demonstrated the greatest improvement in the area of employment; 70 percent of CABG patients compared with 56 percent of transplant patients returned to work approximately one year after surgery. The transplant patients' recovery rate, however, may be more striking considering their preoperative level of impairment.

Comments

Wallwork and Caine note that work status is only one aspect of quality of life and "may not reflect perceived quality-of-life of the patients or other benefits associated with medical care." (See also the discussion of work status in the introduction to these examples on page 13.)

At the one-year follow-up, the investigators found a broad similarity between CABG and transplant surgery patients and the healthy male population within the same age group. Wallwork and Caine emphasize the need for longer-term follow-up of cardiac patients to determine whether improvements reported at one year following surgery are sustained.

Study 8. Cardiac Rehabilitation Programs

Ott, C.R., Sivarajan, E.S., Newton, K.M., Almes, M.J., Bruce, R.A., Bergner, M., and Gilson, B.S. A controlled randomized study of early cardiac rehabilitation: The Sickness Impact Profile as an assessment tool. Heart and Lung 12(2):162-170, 1983.

Key

Technologies Assessed: Cardiac rehabilitation programs
Patient Group: Adults
Diagnosis Type: Acute myocardial infarction (MI)
Measure Category: Physical and psychosocial function
Measures: Sickness Impact Profile (SIP)

Description of Measures

Sickness Impact Profile (SIP). The SIP measures illness-related behavioral dysfunction in 12 areas of living. Ambulation, mobility, and body care and movement comprise the physical dimension. Social interaction, communication, alertness behavior, and emotional behavior represent the psychosocial dimension. Sleep and rest, home maintenance, eating, working, and recreational pastimes comprise the remaining areas. Scores can be calculated for the entire SIP, or they may be separated to isolate the physical or psychosocial dimension.

Purpose of the Study

Ott et al. determined the impact of three different cardiac rehabilitation programs on the quality of life of patients who suffered a myocardial infarction.

Methods

Ott et al. selected 258 MI patients from seven Seattle hospitals and randomly assigned them to one of three rehabilitation groups in a six-month prospective study.

Patients assigned to Group A (control) received conventional medical and nursing management; patients assigned to Group B1 (exercise) participated in an exercise program that continued for three months following discharge; and patients assigned to Group B2 (exercise and teaching/counseling) participated in a teaching and counseling program, in addition to the exercise program of the B1 group. Staff members were blinded to the assignment of exercise patients to groups B1 and B2 until discharge. Patients answered SIP questions pertaining to the week prior to administration to provide baseline data; they were tested again at three months and at the six-month follow-up visit. Changes in SIP scores were calculated by subtracting follow-up scores from the baseline score, which yielded a positive (deterioration), negative (improvement), or no score change.

Results and Conclusions

Ott et al. found that patients who participated in the teaching and counseling program in addition to the exercise program did significantly better than those in the other two groups, particularly in the psychosocial dimension. Patients in the teaching and counseling group also showed an increase in the overall SIP score at the six-month follow-up. In addition, these patients had higher scores in the category of eating, which the investigators attribute to the teaching and counseling sessions that provided information on nutrition and diet.

Comments

The investigators note that their original baseline calculations were faulty, drawn from subjective recollections by patients at the most impaired point of their experience. The investigators also note that the exercise program was an individual, unsupervised program with no peer or counseling support. In spite of these faults, the SIP may be a useful tool in evaluating the recovery progress of patients with myocardial infarctions. Targeting the patients' varying rates of recovery on each of the 12 dimensions measured by the SIP may help clinicians and patients to speed the recovery process in specific areas and to improve the long-term quality of life.

Study 9. Long-term Dialysis and Renal Transplant

Bonney, S., Finkelstein, F.O., Lytton, B., Schiff, M., and Steele, T.E. Treatment of end-stage renal failure in a defined geographic area. Archives of Internal Medicine 138(10):1510-1513, 1978.

Key

Technologies Assessed: Long-term dialysis and renal transplantation
Patient Group: Adults on long-term hemodialysis or transplant recipients
Diagnosis Type: Renal failure

Measure Category: Psychological, physical, and social function
Measures: Quality-of-life indices (work status, sexual functioning), physical activity indices, Kupfer-Detre System Forms 1 and 2

Description of Measures

Quality-of-life indices. These indices included the patients' level of general physical ability, level of sexual function, and current and prior work status.

Physical activity. This was classified according to the functional classifications recommended by the National Kidney Foundation: Class 1, capable of performing all usual types of physical activity; Class 2, unable to perform the most strenuous of usual physical activities; Class 3, unable to perform usual daily physical activities more than occasionally; and Class 4, severe limitation of usual physical activity.

Kupfer-Detre System Form 1 (KDS-1). The KDS-1 evaluates current psychological status.

Kupfer-Detre System Form 2 (KDS-2). The KDS-2 elicits data on the presence or absence of 64 specific physical symptoms.

Purpose of the Study

Bonney et al. determined the impact of long-term hemodialysis and renal transplantation on quality of life.

Methods

Bonney et al. reviewed the medical records of, and conducted structured interviews with, 129 (95 percent of total) long-term home dialysis patients, 23 (82 percent of total) hemodialysis unit patients, and 38 (100 percent of total) patients who received renal transplants between 1967 and 1975 in southern Connecticut. The investigators selected this region because most patients with renal failure were able to receive treatment with a reasonably uniform level of management.

Results and Conclusions

The investigators found that quality of life was lower for dialysis patients than for transplant recipients. The dialysis patients were more likely to be unemployed, to be less physically active, to have less satisfac tory sexual relations, and to suffer from depression, organic brain dysfunction (demonstrated by the KDS-1), and numerous physical complaints (demonstrated by the KDS-2) than patients in the transplant group. Dialysis patients had a mean depression score similar to those of psychiatric outpatients. In contrast, depression scores for the transplant recipients were comparable to those for the general population. Although the transplant patients were generally in better condition physically and mentally than the dialysis patients, they too exhibited manifestations of impaired functioning.

Comments

Data on the quality of life of dialysis and renal transplantation patients may help both patients and physicians consider the impact of these treatments. It may also increase the awareness of the difficulties that may be expected with each course of treatment.

Study 10. Renal Transplantation and Dialysis

Evans, R.W., Manninen, D.L., Garrison, L.P., Jr., Hart, L.G., Blagg, C.R., Gutman, R.A., Hull, A.R., and Lowrie, E.G. The quality of life of patients with end-stage renal disease. New England Journal of Medicine 312(9):553-559, 1985.

Key

Technology Assessed: Renal transplant versus dialysis (home, in-center, and peritoneal)
Patient Group: Adults
Diagnosis Type: End-stage renal disease (ESRD)
Measure Category: Physical, role and social function, and global well-being
Measures: Karnofsky Index, Index of Psychological Affect, Index of Overall Life Satisfaction, Index of Well-Being, work status

Description of Measures

Karnofsky Index. This is an objective measure of overall physical function. Scores range from 1 (moribund) to 10 (normal activity).

Index of Psychological Affect (IPA). The eight bipolar items of the IPA describe respondents' thoughts about their current situation. Responses are averaged to give an overall score ranging from 1 (completely dissatisfied) to 7 (completely satisfied).

Index of Overall Life Satisfaction (IOLS). The bipolar items of the IOLS describe the respondents' overall satisfaction with life. Scoring is similar to that in the IPA.

Index of Well-Being. The Index of Well-Being consists of a combination of responses to the IPA and IOLS. It is weighted toward the former. Scores range from 2.1 (low) to 14.7 (high).

Work status. This measure consists of a response to the question "Are you now able to work for pay full time, part time, or not at all?"

Purpose of the Study

The investigators compared the effectiveness of alternative dialysis methods for ESRD patients using a range of measures related to both clinical status and quality of life.

Methods

Evans et al. compared 859 nonrandomized patients who underwent either renal transplantation or dialysis (home, in-center, or peritoneal). These patients were surveyed from 11 transplantation and dialysis centers nationwide. The investigators analyzed sociodemographic and medical variables as well as the objective and subjective measures of quality of life described above. All data collectors participated in an intensive three-day training session, although much of the training was devoted to medical record abstraction rather than administering quality-of-life instruments. The investigators maintained routine contacts with each center to ensure that uniform procedures were followed. The response rate was over 90 percent.

Results and Conclusions

Evans et al. found that the subjective and objective measures correlated poorly. They found that transplant recipients had the least functional impairment; those treated through in-center dialysis were most impaired. Almost 75 percent of transplant recipients were able to work, compared with 60 percent of those on home dialysis and much lower proportions of the other groups. Case-mix factors, including age, educational level, and comorbidity, had substantial effects on these two measures.

With case-mix adjustment, transplant recipients had the most favorable subjective scores. Younger, more educated, and white patients tended to report higher quality-of-life scores. In contrast to the objective measures, the comorbid conditions studied did not have a significant relation to subjective quality-of-life measures.

The investigators also compared their patients with the general population. Labor-force participation rates showed that end-stage renal disease patients are much less likely to work than is the adult population as a whole. Comparisons of results on the subjective measure to results obtained by Campbell et al. (1976) for the U.S. population showed that "patients with ESRD perceived that they have only a slightly lower quality-of-life than the general population . . . [but] only transplant recipients have a subjective quality-of-life that does not differ significantly from that of the general population." Thus, even with correction for the differences among treatment groups, transplant recipients had consistently higher subjective and objective quality-of-life scores.

Comments

The investigators described some weaknesses in their study, such as the lack of randomization, substantial case-mix variation among treatment groups, a lack of analysis of interaction terms, and no longitudinal data. Nevertheless, the design was strengthened by the training and monitoring of data collectors to promote uniformity, the use of both subjective and objective categories of quality-of-life measures, and the choice of established measures that allow comparisons with other patient groups and with the general population. The low correlation between the objective and subjective indices, observed in a variety of quality-of-life studies, has implications for their use. Subjective measures reveal that these patients may be experiencing levels of quality of life much closer to those of the general population than objective measures might indicate. Although these results may demonstrate the "psychological adaptability" of ESRD patients, and possibly that of chronic disease patients more generally, they also raise policy questions concerning the appropriate standards for treatment decisions.

Study 11. Case Management and Usual and Customary Services for Chronically Mentally Ill Patients

Franklin, J.L., Solovitz, B., Masson, M., Clemons, J.R., and Miller, G.E. An evaluation of case management. American Journal of Public Health 77 (6):674-678, 1987.

Key

Technology Assessed: Case management versus "usual and customary" services for chronically mentally ill patients
Patient Group: Mentally ill adults
Diagnosis Type: Mental illness
Measure Category: Mental, role, and social function
Measures: Social function, Affect Balance Scale, Self-Esteem Scale, Cost-Benefit Analysis

Description of Measures

Social function. A variety of objective and subjective measures were developed to consider six areas: housing, living arrangements, social relations, leisure, income, and employment. The objective measures consisted of quantifiable items in each area; subjective measures were designed to assess satisfaction with conditions in each area. Additionally, an "activities of daily living" measure included self-assessments of performance of such activities as cooking, budgeting, and traveling.

Affect Balance Scale. This assessment measure consists of 10 yes or no items, including a 5-item negative affect scale.

Self-Esteem Scale. This scale includes five statements relating to overall self-esteem, such as "On the whole, I am satisfied with myself," and "I feel useless at times."

Cost-Benefit Analysis. This analysis compared quality-of-life and utilization results with costs incurred by each patient group.

Purpose of the Study

The investigators compared two methods of delivering management and support services to chronically mentally ill patients—"usual and cus tomary" services and a more directed and systematic "case management" approach designed to meet the needs of individual patients.

Methods

Using a randomized, pretest-posttest control-group design, investigators assigned 417 (83 percent) of 500 eligible patients to receive either case management or non-case management services. The investigators reinterviewed 63 percent of the patients one year later.

Results and Conclusions

Patients in the case management group were twice as likely to be readmitted to a mental institution; they stayed longer, incurred higher costs, and used more than twice as many community-based services as the patients in the other group. Investigators found few significant differences in quality-of-life measures between the two groups. They concluded that the experimental case management approach appeared to increase costs substantially without demonstrating any important effect on the quality of life of mental patients. This increase may have resulted from increased detection and correction of an underutilization of services in the experimental group. Furthermore, the one-year time span of the experiment may have been too short to detect significant changes in this chronically ill population.

Comments

The investigators discuss many special considerations required for performing quality-of-life assessments with mentally ill patients, such as difficulties in follow-up. The study also illustrates an outcome contrary to that anticipated by the researchers. They note that case management is "uniformly favored" by professionals to increase effectiveness of services, and they do not advocate any policy conclusions based on their results. Nonetheless, the report provides an example of the use of quality-of-life measures in a context directly related to the evaluation of policies for the delivery of social services, as well as the application of quality-of-life measures to a special patient population.

Study 12. Health Insurance Payment Mechanisms

Brook, R.H., Ware, J.E., Jr., Rogers, W.H., Keeler, E.B., Davies, A.R., Donald, C.A., Goldberg, G.A., Lohr, K.N., Masthay, P.C., and Newhouse, J.P. Does free care improve adults' health? Results from a randomized controlled trial. New England Journal of Medicine 309(23):1426-1434, 1983.

Key

Technology Assessed: Health insurance payment mechanisms
Patient Group: General adult population (under age 65)
Diagnosis Type: None
Measure Category: Physical, mental, social, and global
Measures: General Health Rating Index

Description of Measures

General Health Rating Index (GHRI). The GHRI is completed by patients and consists of the following five categories of items, all scored on 0-100 scales, with higher scores indicating better performance:

(1) Physical Functioning. The 23 items in this category measure personal limitations in self-care, mobility, and physical activities.
(2) Role Functioning. The two role functioning items measure ability to function at work, school, or home.
(3) Social Contacts. These three items measure contact with friends and family during the past month or year.
(4) Mental Health. The 38 mental health items measure anxiety, depression, behavioral and emotional control, and psychological well-being during the previous month.
(5) Health Perception. The 22 items in this category measure the person's perceptions of past, present, and future health; susceptibility to illness; and health concerns.

Purpose of the Study

Brook et al. evaluated whether groups who had access to more health care, through the use of "free" plans in the RAND Health Insurance Experiment, achieved better health status than groups enrolled in a variety of cost-sharing plans.

Methods

A total of 3,958 people, between the ages of 14 and 61 and tested in six study centers, were enrolled in the study for three or five years. All Medicare-eligible patients (for example, the disabled) were excluded. Participants were assigned to a variety of insurance plans; only one of these did not require enrollees to pay a portion of their medical bills. No significant differences between the groups existed at the time of enrollment.

Results and Conclusions

Only role functioning was significantly improved in the free plan. No significant differences were detected among subgroups differing in income and initial health status, but confidence intervals for these groups were wider than those for average enrollees.

Comments

The GHRI was developed for use in a large, controlled trial involving generally healthy adults. Consequently, it provides a well-tested measure for analyzing medical services for broad segments of the population, including individuals who are generally healthy. Adjustments may be necessary for its application to subgroups, such as the poor or elderly, who may have special quality-of-life considerations.

REFERENCES

Bombardier, C., Ware, J., Russell, I.J., Larson, M., Chalmers, A., and Read, J.L. Auranofin therapy and quality of life in patients with rheumatoid arthritis. Results of a multicenter trial. The American Journal of Medicine 81(4):565-578, 1986.

Bonney, S., Finkelstein, F.O., Lytton, B., Schiff, M., and Steele, T.E. Treatment of end-stage renal failure in a defined geographic area. Archives of Internal Medicine 138(10):1510-1513, 1978.

Brook, R.H., Ware, J.E., Jr., Rogers, W.H., Keeler, E.B., Davies, A.R., Donald, C.A., Goldberg, G.A., Lohr, K.N., Masthay, P.C., and Newhouse, J.P. Does free care improve adults' health? Results from a randomized controlled trial. New England Journal of Medicine 309(23):1426-1434, 1983.

Campbell, A., Converse, P.E., and Rodgers, W.L. The Quality of American Life: Perceptions, Evaluations and Satisfactions. New York, Russell Sage Foundation, 1976.

Coates, A., Gebski, V., Bishop, J.F., Jeal, P.N., Woods, R.L., Snyder, R., Tattersall, M.H., Byrne, M., Harvey, V., and Gill, G. Improving the quality of life during chemotherapy for advanced breast cancer. A comparison of intermittent and continuous treatment strategies. New England Journal of Medicine 317(24):1490-1495, 1987.

Croog, S.H., Levine, S., Testa, M.A., Brown, B., Bulpitt, C.J., Jenkins, C.D., Klerman, G.L., and Williams, G.H. The effects of antihypertensive therapy on the quality of life. New England Journal of Medicine 314(26):1657-1664, 1986.

Evans, R.W., Manninen, D.L., Garrison, L.P., Jr., Hart, L.G., Blagg, C.R., Gutman, R.A., Hull, A.R., and Lowrie, E.G. The quality of life of patients with end-stage renal disease. New England Journal of Medicine 312(9):553-559, 1985.

Franklin, J.L., Solovitz, B., Masson, M., Clemons, J.R., and Miller, G.E. An evaluation of case management. American Journal of Public Health 77(6):674-678, 1987.

Hollandsworth, J.G., Jr. Evaluating the impact of medical treatment on the quality of life: A 5-year update. Social Science and Medicine 26(4):425-434, 1988.

Lasry, J.C., Margolese, R.G., Poisson, R., Shibata, H., Fleischer, D., Lafleur, D., Legault, S., and Taillefer, S. Depression and body image following mastectomy and lumpectomy. Journal of Chronic Diseases 40(6):529-534, 1987.

Linn, M.W., Linn, B.S., and Harris, R. Effects of counseling for late stage cancer patients. Cancer 49 (5):1048-1055, 1982.

Meyerowitz, B.W., Sparks, F.C., and Spears, I.K., Adjuvant chemotherapy for breast carcinoma. Cancer 43(5):1613-1618, 1979.

Najman, J.M., and Levine, S. Evaluating the impact of medical care and technologies on the quality of life: A review and critique. Social Science and Medicine [F] 15(2-3):107-115, 1981.

Ott, C.R., Sivarajan, E.S., Newton, K.M., Almes, M.J., Bruce, R.A., Bergner, M., and Gilson, B.S. A controlled randomized study of early cardiac rehabilitation: The Sickness Impact Profile as an assessment tool. Heart and Lung 12(2):162-170, 1983.

Steinberg, M.D., Juliano, M.A., and Wise, L. Psychological outcome of lumpectomy versus mastectomy in the treatment of breast cancer. American Journal of Psychiatry 142(1):34-39, 1985.

Wallwork, J., and Caine, N. A comparison of the quality of life of cardiac transplant patients and coronary artery bypass graft patients before and after surgery. Quality of Life and Cardiovascular Care 1(7) September/October:317-331, 1985.

3

Quality-of-Life Measures in Liver Transplantation

Mark S. Roberts

End-stage liver disease produces substantial changes in the quality of patients' lives. Mental capacities are impaired (in some cases producing coma) by hepatic encephalopathy; large amounts of fluid may accumulate in the abdomen (ascites), with accompanying compromises in mobility, respiration, and increased risk of infection. Increased venous back-pressure produces excessive bleeding in the esophagus and stomach. Decreased liver function may produce serious malnutrition with effects on multiple organ systems.

Therapeutic modalities used to treat these complications often involve trade-offs among many quality-of-life dimensions. For example, venous bypass procedures that lower excessive venous pressure decrease the incidence of bleeding and the amount of ascites, but they may exacerbate hepatic encephalopathy and increase the risk of clotting disorders. When successful, liver transplantation alleviates virtually all of the complications of end-stage liver disease, but it has its own set of effects on a patient's physical well-being and life-style. Although the National Institutes of Health (NIH) Consensus Conference on the evaluation of liver transplantation recommended transplantation as an effective therapeutic modality in certain forms of end-stage liver disease, the report noted: "we

---

Editors' Note: The editors believed it would be instructive to have an article in a field where the quality-of-life work thus far was modest enough to be encompassed in a single short article. Dr. Roberts has prepared such a piece for us in liver transplantation, an area that presents special difficulties for appraisals of quality of life.

lack systematically gathered information on quality of life among longterm survivors" (NIH consensus development statement, 1984).

The following is a brief review of methods that have been used to evaluate the quality of life in liver transplant patients. Standard quality-of-life measures may require the patients to answer many specific and sometimes subtle questions about life-style, as well as the patient's interpretation of the impact of their disease on that life-style. Because patients with end-stage liver disease often have serious cognitive impairments, it is not always possible to use patient-directed, subjective assessment tools.

QUALITY-OF-LIFE MEASURES

A computer-based literature search encompassing medical journals from 1966 to the present, called MEDLINE, produced 13 articles that dealt explicitly with quality-of-life assessment of patients who had survived liver transplantation. The assessment methods used were separated into four categories: alterations in neuropsychiatric and neurophysiologic testing; the rate of return to work, school, or prior social situation; the presence or absence of psychopathology; and scores on specifically designed quality-of-life measures.

Alterations in Neuropsychiatric Testing

In a study of liver transplant candidates, Guthkelch et al. (1979) showed that patients with end-stage liver disease exhibit significant abnormalities on several neurophysiologic tests, including visual evoked potentials and brain stem-evoked potentials even in the absence of clinical encephalopathy. Sclabassi et al. (1983), working with a group of 170 transplant candidates, demonstrated that the severity of these abnormalities correlated with the severity of clinical encephalopathy, when alterations in mental functioning were apparent on examination. Hegedus et al. (1984) found that these abnormalities and associated neuropsychiatric impairments in memory, visual-spatial awareness and perception, and cognitive capability persisted after transplantation and that they had a detrimental impact on patients' activities of daily living.

More extensive testing was performed on a subset of the patients mentioned above. In a prospective analysis of 15 patients tested on 30 separate measures of intelligence, memory, language, and other neuropsychiatric functions both before and six weeks after transplantation, Tar

tar et al. (1983, 1984) found no difference between these patients' scores on the Minnesota Multiphasic Personality Inventory (MMPI), 16 Personality Factor Questionnaire (16PF), and standard intelligence quotient (IQ) tests and a matched group of patients suffering from Crohn's disease, another chronic liver disorder. There were, however, significant improvements in scores on the Sickness Impact Profile.

Ability to Return to Work, School, or Prior Social Situation

Among a group of transplant patients surviving more than one year, Starzl et al. (1979) measured improvements in the quality of life by noting whether the patient returned to school or work. The investigators found improvements in 22 of 26 pediatric and adult patients. In a consecutive series of 70 transplant patients, Williams et al. (1987) devised a simple three-level scale indicating full, partial, or no rehabilitation, depending upon whether the patient had returned to work or school, was able to leave the hospital and live at home, or exhibited no improvement in function. Full rehabilitation was achieved by 30 percent to 50 percent of the sample, and the likelihood of success was found to correlate with pretransplant condition: the sicker the patient was prior to surgery, the less likely the patient was to achieve full rehabilitation. Among 18 long-term survivors of 94 transplants, Macdougall et al. (1980) found 2 patients who demonstrated "improvement" through their return to work.

More recently, as part of a larger prospective study of 65 transplant patients given questionnaires six months before and at least six months after transplant, Tartar et al. (1988) reported significant improvements in several measures assumed to be correlated with quality of life. These measures included return to work or school, number of days spent in the hospital, exercise tolerance, and financial status.

Presence of Psychopathology

In a description of detailed posttransplant psychiatric interviews with patients who were well enough both before and after the transplant to sustain a two to two and one-half hour interview, House et al. (1983) noted an increased incidence of depression, anxiety, regression, dependence, and anger, as well as eight other psychological conditions. Only the incidence of organic brain syndrome, presumably related to the poor metabolic milieu, decreased after transplantation.

Scores on Specific Quality-of-Life Questionnaires

Tymstra et al. (1986) developed a three-level questionnaire indicating serious, not serious, and no physical complaints and high, moderate, and low global life satisfaction. Two observers scored the questionnaire for eight transplant survivors. Seven of eight patients reported high or moderate satisfaction; five of eight reported either no serious complaints or no complaints. Zitelli et al. (1987) evaluated several measures in 90 consecutive pediatric patients who survived transplantation. Quality-of-life measures included the number of hospitalizations and hospital days, the age-appropriateness of year in school, cognitive functioning, and multiple measures of behavioral adjustment. The average number of days spent in the hospital decreased by 22 days each year, 75 percent of the pediatric patients exhibited increased growth rates, and 78 percent of patients were found to be no more than one year behind their age-appropriate grade level. A unique aspect of this study involved the administration of a quality-of-life questionnaire to the *parents* of the child, concerning motor skills, school and home behavior, and relationships with parents and siblings. Each question was scored on a five-point scale. Many patients improved an average of one to two points after transplantation.

The 1988 study by Tartar et al. described above also stressed performance on several quality-of-life measures, both from the patients' and families' perspective. The investigators reported substantial improvements in the responses on the Sickness Impact Profile, the Social Behavior Assessment Schedule, and several psychological instruments designed to measure family health and mechanisms for coping with stress.

CONCLUSIONS

A major difficulty in evaluating the effect of liver transplantation on the quality of life of patients suffering from end-stage liver disease is the inability of many pretransplant patients to complete evaluations that could then be compared with posttransplantation scores. Such profound impairments of mental capacity in end-stage liver disease mean that a large percentage of transplantation candidates cannot be evaluated by standard quality-of-life measures that rely solely on subjective patient responses. To circumvent this difficulty, several investigators have used measurable, neurophysiologic tests that they believe correlate with the degree of mental impairment as a proxy for quality of life. The assumption is that mental impairment itself implies a poor quality of life. Similarly, several researchers have used the level of general function, measured by return to the work, school, or social position occupied before developing liver disease, as estimates of quality of life.

Under the assumption that quality of life is a subjective, individual perception of the value of a health state, we cannot expect validity in a measure of quality of life taken when a patient's mental capacity is impaired. Nevertheless, this review supports several statements regarding the quality of life following liver transplantation.

First, measurements of the return to work or social position are, in general, reliable, easy to measure, and, all else held equal, must at least be positively correlated with quality of life. (See the cautionary remarks on this issue on page 13).

Second, because of mental impairment, coma, or severity of illness, the decision to transplant is often made not by the patient, but rather by the patient's family and physicians when the patient is deemed incompetent to assess the risks and benefits. Therefore, the development of measures of level of mental functioning, return to work, and the presence or absence of mental illness may help the family make more informed decisions regarding the best therapeutic intervention for the patient. In these circumstances we must rely more heavily on clinical testing or on ratings assumed to be proxies for quality of life.

Third, when the liver disease is not sufficiently advanced to produce serious mental impairment, there is substantial evidence that several self-and family-reported quality-of-life measures will show improvement over the pretransplant state, but quality of life may not return to the level the patient enjoyed prior to the development of liver disease.

REFERENCES

Guthkelch, A.N., Sclabassi, R.J., Van Thiel, D.H., Schade, R.R., Hirsch, R.P., and Starzl, T.E. A preliminary review of neurophysiological data in patients evaluated for liver transplantation. (Abstract) Hepatology 3(5):827, 1979.

Hegedus, A.M., Tartar, R.E., Van Thiel, D.H., Gavaler, J.S., Schade, R.R., and Starzl, T.E. Neuropsychiatric status of liver transplantation patients one year after successful liver transplantation. (Abstract) Hepatology 4(5):1085, 1984.

House, R., Dubovsky, S.L., and Penn, I. Psychiatric aspects of hepatic transplantation. Transplantation 36(2):146-150, 1983.

Macdougall, B.R., Calne, R.Y., McMaster, P., and Williams, R. Survival and rehabilitation after orthotopic liver transplantation. Lancet 1(8182):1326-1328, 1980.

National Institutes of Health (NIH) consensus development statement: Liver transplantation-- June 20-23, 1983. Hepatology 4(1):107s-110s (Supplement), 1984.

Sclabassi, R.J., Guthkelch, A.N., Van Thiel, D.H., Schade, R.R., Hirsch, R.P., and Starzl, T.E. Neuropsychological assessment of liver transplant candidates. (Abstract) Hepatology 3 (5):120, 1983.

Starzl, T.E., Koep, L.J., Schröter, G.P., Hood, J., Halgrimson, C.G., Porter, K.A., and Weill, R., 3rd. The quality of life after liver transplantation. Transplantation Proceedings 11(1):252-256, 1979.

Tartar, R.E., Hegedus, A.M., Gavaler, J.S.J., Schade, R.R., Van Thiel, D.H., and Starzl, T.E. Acute effects of liver transplantation on neuropsychological capacity as determined by studies performed pretransplantation and four to six weeks following surgery. (Abstract) Hepatology 3(5):830, 1983.

Tartar, R.E., Van Thiel, D.H., Hegedus, A.M., Schade, R.R., Gavaler, J.S., and Starzl, T.E. Neuropsychiatric status after liver transplantation. Journal of Laboratory and Clinical Medicine 103(5):776-782, 1984.

Tartar, R.E., Erb, S., Biller, P.A., Switala, J., and Van Thiel, D.H. The quality of life following liver transplantation: A preliminary report. Gastroenterology Clinics of North America 17 (1):207-217, 1988.

Tymstra, T., Bucking, J., Roorda, J., van den Heuvel, W.J., and Gips, C.H. The psychosocial impact of a liver transplant programme. Liver 6(5):302-309, 1986.

Williams, J.W., Vera, S., and Evans, L.S. Socioeconomic aspects of hepatic transplantation. American Journal of Gastroenterology 82(11):1115-1119, 1987.

Zitelli, B.J., Gartner, J.C., Malatack, J.J., Urbach, A.H., Miller, J.W., Williams, L., Kirkpatrick, B., Breinig, M.K., and Ho, M. Pediatric liver transplantation: Patient evaluation and selection, infectious complications, and life-style after transplantation. Transplantation Proceedings 19(4):3309-3316, 1987.

4

Quality-of-Life Measures and Methods Used to Study Antihypertensive Medications

Sol Levine and Sydney H. Croog

Several objectives and concerns guided our selection of instruments to measure the effects of antihypertensive medication on the quality of life of patients (Croog et al. 1986). Our study was based on a randomized double-blind clinical trial of a relatively large population dispersed in 30 centers throughout the country. Hence, we wished to obtain measures that were valid and objective and could be administered in a rigorous, standardized manner in many different settings. We sought to obtain instruments that could be administered in a relatively brief time, and, as far as possible, had already demonstrated their usefulness in other studies.

Other considerations involved our conception of the measurement of quality of life as a construct. Measures of quality of life necessarily must be modified by the severity and course or trajectory of the illness or condition, as well as the social and demographic characteristics of the individual and the social context in which he or she lives (Croog and Levine 1989). Because we were studying hypertensive patients whose modes of life approximate those of otherwise healthy persons in most respects, we needed to obtain a comprehensive picture of the profile of the patient's life that would be very similar to that of a nonhypertensive, healthy person. If we were studying the quality of life of patients with chronic obstructive pulmonary disease, we would have modified our measures and selected a more constricted band of indicators. Or, if we

---

Editors' Note: The editors invited the authors to describe how they went about choosing quality-of-life measures in their research on antihypertensive medications. We also asked the authors to add any advice they cared to give others.

were measuring the quality of life of a terminally ill patient, we would have focused on how well the person could interact with others, recognize others, derive some satisfaction from seeing friends or relatives, and the like. We obviously would not focus in a significant way upon the terminally ill person's ability to carry out activities in the community.

For our study of hypertensive patients, we selected measures in line with the conception that five major dimensions of quality of life must be assessed (Levine and Croog 1984). The first area for assessment was the performance of social roles, including those of spouse, parent, worker, friend, and community citizen. A second major dimension was the physiological state of the individual. The third was the emotional state of the individual; the fourth, the intellective or cognitive functioning status of the individual; and fifth, a general sense of well-being and life satisfaction.

Among possible measures, the RAND General Well-Being Scale first met our requirements (Brook et al. 1979). It consists of 22 self-administered questions that comprise six subscales assessing anxiety, depression, general health, positive well-being, self-control, and vitality. This scale has a long history, has been used extensively in the large RAND Health Insurance study, and has proven its usefulness. For the purposes of further measuring emotional status, we used a series of subscales from the Brief Symptom Inventory (BSI), developed by Derogatis and Spencer (1982). The BSI is a 53-item, self-report inventory designed to assess the psychological symptom patterns of respondents.

In measuring cognitive or intellective functioning, we used two tests that are among the most established and widely used in the field: the Visual Reproduction Test of the Wechsler Memory Scale (Wechsler 1945, Wechsler and Stone 1973), and the Reitan Trail-Making Test (Reitan 1958). The Visual Reproduction Test assesses neuropsychological function on the basis of diagram images, and the Trail-Making Test measures visual-motor speed and integration.

Selecting instruments for use in the study of hypertensive patients was complicated because existing scales and measures were not directly pertinent to this population for some dimensions of quality of life. Hence, it was necessary to adapt existing instruments for the special needs of this study and, in some instances, to construct new measures.

To assess physical symptoms associated with antihypertensive medications, we adapted questions used commonly in clinical practice, framing these as a Physical Symptoms Distress Index (Hypertension Detection and Follow-up Program Cooperation Group 1982, Derogatis and Spencer

1982). Because sexual dysfunction may be an important side effect in pharmacologic treatment of hypertensives, we developed a four-item index suited for the survey research approach in this study, the Sexual Symptoms Distress Index. It was adapted from previous work (Hogan et al. 1980, Derogatis and Spencer 1982). Measures of life satisfaction were based, in part, on scales from items employed by Campbell et al. (1976) in a study of quality of life, and in part on research by Haynes et al. (1978a,b) on stress and heart disease within the Framingham Heart Study. To assess changes in work performance that might be associated with antihypertensive medications, we employed a number of items concerning work performance, adapted in part from previous scale items by House (1981).

If we were carrying out this study again, we would probably follow a similar program in selecting instruments for assessing quality-of-life dimensions. The measures would be adapted, of course, for the particular illness condition being studied because it is necessary to select a range or band of indicators specifically appropriate for the health condition under consideration. We would certainly select shorter, generic, or fewer scales when this could be done without sacrificing validity and reliability. Insofar as possible, we would employ widely used, standardized measures. We would again use the RAND General Well-Being Scale.

In studying cognitive function, we would employ a broader range of measures than we did in our previous study of hypertensive men, selecting tests that might be somewhat more sensitive to the effects of antihypertensive medications on cognitive function. We would select tests that would be less subject to the learning effect imposed by repeated experience, such as those employing digits or nonsense syllables. In short, we would employ a brief version of our total instrument, although we have some reservations about how far we should go in shortening some of the scales. Finally, we would explore the possibilities of using computer-assisted methods in carrying out at least part of the data collection, although there are many advantages to having interviewers control the administration of the questionnaire as a whole.

REFERENCES

Brook, R.H., Rogers, W.H., Williams, K.N., Ware, J.E., Jr., Stewart, A.L., Johnston, S.A., and Donald, C.A. Conceptualization and Measurement of Health for Adults in the Health Insurance Study. Vol. III. Mental Health. R-1987/3-HEW. Santa Monica, California, The RAND Corporation, 1979.

Campbell, A., Converse, P.E., and Rodgers, W.L. The Quality of American Life: Perceptions, Evaluations, and Satisfactions. New York, Russell Sage Foundation, 1976.

Croog, S.H., and Levine, S. Quality of life and health care interventions. In Freedman, H.E., and Levine, S., eds. The Handbook of Medical Sociology, Fourth Edition. Englewood Cliffs, New Jersey, Prentice Hall, 1989.

Croog, S.H., Levine, S., Testa, M.A., Brown. B., Bulpitt, C.J., Jenkins, C.D., Klerman, G.L., and Williams, G.H. The effects of antihypertensive therapy on the quality of life. New England Journal of Medicine 314(26):1657-1664, 1986.

Derogatis, L.R., and Spencer, P.M. The Brief Symptom Inventory (BSI), Administration, Scoring and Procedures Manual 1. Baltimore, Johns Hopkins University School of Medicine (privately printed), 1982.

Haynes, S.G., Levine, S., Scotch, N., Feinleib, M., and Kannel, W.B. The relationship of psychosocial factors to coronary heart disease in the Framingham study. I. Methods and risk factors. American Journal of Epidemiology 107(5):362-383, 1978a.

Haynes, S.G., Feinleib, M., Levine, S., Scotch, N., and Kannel, W.B. The relationship of psychosocial factors to coronary heart disease in the Framingham study. II. Prevalence of coronary heart disease. American Journal of Epidemiology 107(5):384-402, 1978b.

Hogan, M.J., Wallin, J.D., and Baer, R.M. Antihypertensive therapy and male sexual dysfunction. Psychosomatics 21(3):236-237, 1980.

House, J.S. Work Stress and Social Support. Reading, Massachusetts, Addison-Wesley, 1981.

Hypertension Detection and Follow-up Program Cooperation Group. The effect of treatment on mortality in "mild" hypertension: Results of the Hypertension Detection and Follow-up Program. New England Journal of Medicine 307(16):976-980, 1982.

Levine, S., and Croog, S.H. What constitutes quality of life? A conceptualization of the dimensions of life quality in healthy populations and patients with cardiovascular disease. In Wenger, N.K., Mattson, M.E., Furberg, C.D., and Elinson, J., eds. Assessment of Quality of Life in Clinical Trials of Cardiovascular Therapies. New York, Le Jacq Publishing, Inc., 46-58, 1984.

Reitan, R.M. Trail-Making Manual for Administration, Scoring, and Interpretation. Department of Neurology, Section of Neuropsychology, Indiana University Medical Center, Indianapolis, 1958.

Wechsler, D. A standardized memory scale for clinical use. Journal of Psychology 19:87-95, 1945.

Wechsler, D., and Stone, C.P. Instruction Manual for the Wechsler Memory Scale. New York, The Psychological Corporation, 1973.

5

The Use of Quality-of-Life Measures in the Private Sector

Bryan R. Luce, Joan M. Weschler, and Carol Underwood

This chapter explores industry's use of the quality-of-life concept, how it is applied, and the expected outcomes of its use. Although we emphasize the private sector, most published accounts to date have been supported by the public sector, usually funded by government agencies through universities. As discussed below, this trend may be changing.

As our references show, the published and fugitive literature indicates wide-ranging interest in quality-of-life measures. Although only a few studies funded by companies in the private sector have been published, most pharmaceutical companies are at least entertaining the idea of incorporating such measures into future clinical trials. Some have made the explicit decision to use them in all clinical trials.

The belief in the importance of quality-of-life measures in the assessment of palliative drugs appears to be well entrenched. The extent of the use of these scales is not yet reflected in the literature because of the time lag between the conduct of clinical trials and the publication of results. Our findings indicate that it is reasonable to anticipate an increase in the number of companies that use such scales, an observation that will soon be manifested in the literature.

METHOD OF STUDY

To assess the use of quality-of-life measures by the private sector, we devised a three-part study. First, we conducted a literature review to provide background information on the field, as well as to search for private-sector studies that incorporated these measures. Second, we developed and distributed a questionnaire to ask private pharmaceutical and device companies about their current and prospective uses of quality-of-life instruments in clinical trials. Third, we conducted interviews with officials at the Food and Drug Administration (FDA), other government agencies, and private companies to ascertain their respective positions on the salience, validity, and usefulness of these measures. Our ultimate objective was to identify groups that are using, or plan to use, quality-of-life measures and to determine why they are using them.

Private-Sector Research in Quality of Life

In 1986, published research revealed for the first time that not only were private companies interested in quality-of-life assessment, but also that they were funding quality-of-life studies as part of their clinical trials. In an article published by the *New England Journal of Medicine*, Croog et al. (1986) reported that, in a randomized double-blind clinical trial, patients who took the oral antihypertensive pharmaceutical agent captopril enjoyed a higher quality of life than those taking propranolol or methyldopa. Specifically, patients who took captopril, as compared with patients who took methyldopa, "scored significantly higher on measures of general well-being, had fewer side effects, and had better scores for work performance, visual-motor functioning, and measures of life satisfaction." Patients who took propranolol experienced intermediate well-being compared with that when they took the two other agents.

A few months later, Bombardier et al. (1986) published in *The American Journal of Medicine* the results of a clinical trial that assessed the effects of auranofin, a pharmaceutical agent used to treat rheumatoid arthritis, on patients' quality of life. In a double-blind study at 14 centers, the effects of auranofin were compared with those of a placebo in the treatment of patients with classic or definite rheumatoid arthritis. The auranofin group, as a whole, experienced relatively higher frequencies of adverse effects, but such events were usually mild and transient. More importantly, from the investigators' point of view, a greater proportion of the auranofin-treated patients than of the placebo-treated patients reported a "marked improvement" in their mobility, including their ability to walk, climb stairs, and raise unaided from a sitting position.

These studies are important for several reasons. First, they indicate that quality-of-life measures are considered an increasingly important part of clinical trials, despite the lack of consensus on the meaning and operationalization of this concept. Second, they reinforce the argument favoring an increased role for quality-of-life considerations in clinical decisionmaking. Finally, they suggest that quality-of-life studies have potential marketing value.

Food and Drug Administration Perspective

Quality of life is a widely discussed concept that elicits a variety of opinions. Its relative utility is debated by researchers in the field. Investigators who use quality-of-life measures clearly believe they are a valuable tool. Others, however, contend that they seem to be indistinguishable from other measures routinely used to assess drug safety and efficacy. Indeed, in the course of several interviews, officials at the FDA suggested that quality-of-life instruments have as their focus aspects of tests already in use to target side effects. In other words, they believe that these measures are not particularly new but have merely been placed under a new rubric.

The FDA has no specific quality-of-life regulatory requirements, in large part because the agency believes that the research community that has developed and refined quality-of-life scales has not been able to show unequivocally that the instruments are "sufficiently credible." As one FDA official noted, highly refined measures are required to differentiate the effects of a drug from the effects of the disease it is meant to treat. Nevertheless, FDA officials express interest in better understanding quality of life, although they consider the state of the art too immature to warrant mandatory inclusion in clinical trials.

This is not to suggest that the FDA has entirely dismissed quality of life as a potentially important factor in clinical trials. One FDA official noted that the usefulness of these measures lies in the attention given to the "downside" of drugs. Although side effects have been recorded, the broader notion of impact on a person's life has not been studied. Quality-of-life scales could be useful, he continued, if they were refined to detect subtle distinctions among pharmaceutical agents. (This view can be contrasted with the findings of the reports given as examples in Chapter 2.)

Thus, although the FDA seems to be interested in the concept, it remains unconvinced of its ultimate validity. The results of our survey of pharmaceutical companies (see discussion that follows) suggest, nevertheless, that there is a perceived advantage to incorporating quality-of-life measurement in clinical drug trials; it is thought to increase the likelihood of FDA approval. Some workers in this field believe that the FDA has actually mandated the use of such studies.*

The FDA is closely monitoring the use of quality-of-life measures in clinical trials and the incorporation of quality-of-life claims in advertising and comparative claims. Pharmaceutical companies often make such claims to try to show that their product has fewer adverse side effects than those of their competitors. Although pharmaceutical companies are allowed to incorporate these claims on their labels, they must present well-supported data. The FDA is particularly skeptical of vague claims and has objected in the past to assertions that a drug is "patient-friendly."

Private Industry Perspective

Some spokespersons in the private sector were forthcoming in responding to questions about their use of quality-of-life instruments in clinical trials; others were reluctant, a result of the highly competitive nature of private industry. Based on informal and formal conversations with research scientists at several pharmaceutical companies, we determined that researchers in the private sector share a general interest in the use of these measures in clinical trials. The next four to five years are expected to produce a proliferation of the use of quality-of-life instruments to support claims that one drug is superior to another in this important respect. We also detected a sense among individuals in private industry that consumers as well as physicians show a growing interest in, and awareness of, the various effects of medications on life quality. For these reasons, many private pharmaceutical companies have made the explicit decision to use quality-of-life measures in clinical trials.

In an interview with one industry spokesperson, we learned that their research scientists are currently using quality-of-life instruments in clinical trials of several drugs developed to palliate the symptoms of chronic diseases. He reported further that company research scientists have made an explicit clinical policy decision to consider quality-of-life components in all clinical trials. He stated that the emphasis on quality of life comes from cost-containment considerations, the need for third-party cost justification, and from competition among similar agents. He believes that

---

* FDA officials have not indicated that quality-of-life studies are required for premarket approval. Nevertheless, Battelle is conducting a quality-of-life study and is about to begin another at the time of this writing. Both are part of Phase III clinical trials. The FDA has reportedly requested that the company submit quality-of-life data.

quality-of-life measures allow the company to demonstrate that their product is superior to another similar agent in the traditional market.

RESULTS OF THE QUALITY-OF-LIFE SURVEY

In cooperation with the Pharmaceutical Manufacturers Association (PMA) and the Health Industry Manufacturers Association (HIMA), Battelle conducted a survey of pharmaceutical and medical companies to determine how widely quality-of-life instruments are being used in the private sector. Both the PMA and HIMA agreed to send Battelle's survey questionnaire to a subset of their respective memberships.

The questionnaire was designed to produce an estimate of the number of companies that have used or are currently using quality-of-life instruments in the conduct of their clinical trials of drugs and devices and to learn whether they plan to continue using them. The questionnaire also probes the reasons companies are or are not using these instruments and asks what types of specific instruments are being used.

Pharmaceutical Industry

The Pharmaceutical Manufacturers Association sent the Battelle questionnaire to a total of 61 pharmaceutical companies, representing approximately two-thirds of its membership. Thirty-four companies (56 percent) responded to the questionnaire. Highlights of the results are presented in Table 5-1.

Of the 34 companies responding, 21 (62 percent) reported they have used some type of quality-of-life instrument in their clinical trials of drugs. All but one reported they are currently using such instruments.

In this survey, the two most frequently cited reasons for using quality-of-life instruments in clinical trials are marketing considerations and internal management or clinical decisionmaking. One company pointed out that quality-of-life measurement is one way to help determine a drug's efficacy when a complicated disease state is present. About one-half of the companies believe that the likelihood of FDA approval will be increased if such measures are used. Some report that quality-of-life studies are required for FDA approval, although this may be a misperception. Somewhat less than one-half of the companies consider having publications in scientific journals an important reason to conduct these studies.

The pharmaceutical companies represented in this sample are using several other instruments in addition to the general, standardized research

TABLE 5-1 Highlights of Survey Results on Quality-of-Life Measurement by Pharmaceutical Firms

Company Activity	Total Number of Companies	Number Reporting	Percent
Companies Using Quality-of-Life Instruments			
Have used	34	21	62
Are currently using	34	20	59
Reasons for use	21		
1. Marketing considerations		15	71
2. Internal management/clinical decisionmaking		13	62
3. Increased likelihood of FDA approval		10	48
4. Publications in scientific journals		8	38
5. FDA requirements for approval		4	19
Standardized instruments used	21		
1. General Health Rating Index (GHRI)		4	19
2. Quality of Well-Being (QWB) Index		3	14
3. General Well-Being (GWB) Index		3	14
4. Nottingham Health Profile (NHP)		3	14
5. Sickness Impact Profile (SIP)		2	10
6. McMaster Health Index		2	10
Developed own quality-of-life instrument(s)	21	14	67
Specific to drug	14	11	79
Both general and specific		5	36
Criteria used in selecting quality-of-life instrument(s)	21		
Validity		18	86
Reliability		16	76
Sensitivity		15	71
Specificity		12	57
Length		13	62
Comprehensiveness		11	52
Cost		9	43
Will continue to use quality-of-life instruments		21	100
Companies Not Using Quality-of-Life Instruments			
Have never used	34	13	38
Reasons for nonuse	13		
1. Not relevant		6	46
2. Too expensive		1	8
3. Not aware of instruments		1	8

Company Activity	Total Number of Companies	Number Reporting	Percent
Will use in future	13	9	69
Reasons	9		
1. Marketing considerations		9	100
2. Increased likelihood of FDA approval		9	100
3. Publications in scientific journals		7	78
4. Internal management/ clinical decisionmaking		5	56
5. FDA requirements for approval		2	22

NOTE: Surveys were sent to 61 companies; 34 responded.

tools we listed in our survey (see Table 5-1). Although each of these all also use other quality-of-life scales. Among those listed are the Beck Depression Inventory, Dupuy Life Satisfaction, Wechsler Memory Scale, Fleming Self-Esteem Hospital Anxiety and Depression Scale, and Women's Health Questionnaire.

Fourteen (67 percent) companies have developed their own quality-of-life instruments, and the majority of these have been specific to the drug or disease state under consideration. In our survey, the greatest number of instruments developed by the companies themselves pertained to heart disease, hypertension, and congestive heart failure. Companies also mentioned that they had designed scales related to sexual dysfunction, gastrointestinal disorders, and cancer.

Criteria used to select or develop a quality-of-life measure—including validity, reliability, sensitivity, specificity, and length—are cited by at least half of the companies surveyed that have used such measures. Less than half (43 percent) of the companies acknowledged cost as a criterion. Also listed as important considerations were ease of administration and scoring, simplicity and time of administration, and the need to evaluate the patient's cognitive state.

Of the 34 companies responding to the questionnaire, 13 have never used a quality-of-life instrument in their clinical trials. Nine (69 percent) of these companies, however, report that they plan to use them in the future; four (31 percent) do not. The most frequently cited reason for not using these instruments is that they are not relevant to the particular drug or disease state.

Several respondents commented that, until recently, quality-of-life studies have simply not been an issue in certain therapeutic areas or have not been considered necessary to confirm efficacy and safety. Only one respondent cited cost as a reason for not sponsoring such studies. Most of the companies in this group cited marketing considerations and increased likelihood of FDA approval as reasons for using such instruments in the future. Over half included publications in scientific journals as a reason. A few respondents anticipate increased attention to quality-of-life studies from the FDA (one company mentioned oncology specifically).

Medical Device Companies

The Health Industry Manufacturers Association (HIMA) sent Battelle's questionnaire to a sample of 25 member companies. This sample was selected by HIMA's Health Care Financing Committee and is considered to be representative of their membership as a whole.

Only six medical device companies responded to the questionnaire, and only one reported using quality-of-life instruments in their clinical trials of devices. Two companies said that they plan to use them in the future, and three do not. Reasons cited for not using such instruments are that they are not relevant or the company has not been aware of them.

A second mailing conducted by HIMA yielded no additional responses from the sample of medical device companies. That three-quarters of the medical device companies did not respond to the questionnaire suggests low salience and sparse usage of quality-of-life instruments in the device sector, especially compared with the drug sector.

CONCLUSIONS

Quality-of-life instruments are being more widely used and more thoroughly debated than ever before. The industry-wide trend to use these measures in clinical trials has been noticeable during the past three years. Researchers in the field expect this trend to continue to be strong and that, ultimately, usage will become routine. These studies can be expected to continue to gain importance in the coming years, both in the public and private sectors and in assessing the comparative effects of different medical interventions on patients. Therefore, instruments designed to measure quality of life will be subjected to increasingly sophisticated refinement and elaboration, even as the theoretical debate about the meaning of quality of life persists. The continued emphasis on, and development of, quality-of-life instruments can be expected to have significant marketing value for the private sector and to contribute to more humane health care services.

Nevertheless, because it is difficult to grasp a complex concept and even more challenging to capture it in a measurement instrument, disagreements will persist about quality of life and its quantification. This ongoing struggle with the concept of quality of life and its ramifications should continue to prove fruitful.

REFERENCES

Bombardier, C., Ware, J., Russell, I.J., Larson, M., Chalmers, A., and Read, J.L. Auranofin therapy and quality of life in patients with rheumatoid arthritis. Results of a multicenter trial. The American Journal of Medicine 81(4):565-578, 1986.

Croog, S.H., Levine, S., Testa, M.A., Brown, B., Bulpitt, C.J., Jenkins, C.D., Klerman, G.L., and Williams, G.H. The effects of antihypertensive therapy on the quality of life. New England Journal of Medicine 314(26):1657-1664, 1986.

SELECTED FURTHER READING

Anderson, J.P., Bush, J.W., and Berry, C.C. Classifying function for health outcome and quality of life evaluation. Medical Care 24(5):454-469, 1986.

Berkman, L.F., and Syme, S.L. Social networks, host resistance, and mortality: A nine-year follow-up study of Alameda County Residents. American Journal of Epidemiology 109(2):186-204, 1979.

de Haes, J.C., and Welvaart, K. Quality of life after breast cancer surgery. Journal of Surgical Oncology 28(2):123-125, 1985.

Evans, R. W., Manninen, D.L., Garrison, L.P., Jr., Hart, L.G., Blagg, C.R., Gutman, R.A., Hull, A.R., and Lowrie, E.G. The quality of life of patients with end-stage renal disease. New England Journal of Medicine 312(9):553-559, 1985.

Kutner, N.G., Brogan, D., and Kutner, M.H. End-stage renal disease treatment modality and patients' quality of life. American Journal of Nephrology 6(5):396-402, 1986.

Lasry, J.C., Margolese, R.G., Poisson, R., Shibata, H., Fleischer, D., Lafleur, D., Legault, S., and Taillefer, S. Depression and body image following mastectomy and lumpectomy. Journal of Chronic Diseases 40(6):529-534, 1987.

Levine, S., and Croog, S.H. What constitutes quality of life? A conceptualization of the dimensions of life quality in healthy populations and patients with cardiovascular disease. In Wenger, N.K., Mattson, M.E., Furberg, C.D., and Elinson, J., eds. Assessment of Quality of Life in Clinical Trials of Cardiovascular Therapies. New York, Le Jacq Publishing, Inc., 1984.

Morris, J.N., and Sherwood, S. Quality of life of cancer patients at different stages in the disease trajectory. Journal of Chronic Diseases 40(6):545-556, 1987.

Priestman, T.J., and Baum, M. Evaluation of quality of life in patients receiving treatment for advanced breast cancer. Lancet 1(7965):899-900, 1976.

Schipper, H., and Levitt, M. Measuring quality of life: Risks and benefits. Cancer Treatment Reports 69(10):11-16, 1985.

Schuessler, K.F., and Fisher, G.A. Quality of life research and sociology. Annual Review of Sociology 11:129-149, 1985.

Siegrist, J. Impaired quality of life as a risk factor in cardiovascular disease. Journal of Chronic Diseases 40(6):571-578, 1987.

Spitzer, W.O., Dobson, A.J., Hall, J., Chesterman, E., Levi, J., Shepherd, R., Battista, R.N., and Catchlove, B.R. Measuring the quality of life of cancer patients: A concise QL-index for use by physicians. Journal of Chronic Diseases 34(12):585-597, 1981.

Troidl, H., Kusche, J., Vestweber, K.H., Eypasch, E., Koeppen, L., and Bouillon, B. Quality of life: An important endpoint both in surgical practice and research. Journal of Chronic Diseases 40(6):523-528, 1987.

World Health Organization. Constitution of the World Health Organization. In: Basic Documents. Geneva, WHO, 1947.

6

Assessing Quality of Life: Measures and Utility

J. Ivan Williams and Sharon Wood-Dauphinee

Quality-of-life research has included the study of levels of economic, political, social, and psychological well-being resulting from varying governmental and economic systems, as well as policies and public programs related to health. Schuessler and Fisher (1985) wrote that quality-of-life research began in the 1960s with the *Report of the President's Commission on National Goals in the United States.* Most specialists agree that the term "quality" has the same meaning as "grade" or "rank," which can range from high to low or best to worst.

What elements of life are to be so graded? The units of analysis can be as large as a nation. Countries can be ranked on their economic systems and on the types and amounts spent by governments on social programs relative to expenditures on industry and the military. At the level of the individual, the elements can be objective (for example, job, income, shelter, and food) or subjective (happiness, sense of well-being, self-realization and the perceptions of the worth and value of life, and the like).

Editors' Note: The authors have supplied information about sources of descriptions of measures and their validity and reliability. Those especially concerned about such matters may wish to go directly to the section entitled "Strategies Used to Assess Instruments," and then to the section entitled "Three Sources of Descriptive Information for Quality-of-Life Measures," which lists three key reference works that provide names, descriptions, and properties of a number of standard instruments. Readers may then skip to "Ten Review Forms for Quality-of-Life Measures," where sources are listed and review forms supplied for some instruments not described in standard works. This chapter contains a special segment that describes utility analysis, a special econometric approach to measures of quality of life.

The best known studies of the quality of life of individuals are those of Andrews and Witney (1976) and Campbell and colleagues (1976, 1980) at the Institute for Social Research at the University of Michigan. Both teams of investigators asked questions about the domains of life satisfaction, including work, marriage, leisure activities, family, housing, and neighborhood. They developed a global measure of satisfaction by combining the scores in a general measure.

Quality of life studies in the health sector are more limited in scope. In the health sciences, the task at hand is to assess the impact of disease and its management, including interventions, on the well-being of the patient. The health states of the individuals may influence their quality of life without determining it. As Ware (1987) noted "jobs, housing, schools, and the neighborhood are not attributes of an individual's health, and they are well outside the purview of the health care system."

Health care researchers have developed numerous measures of quality of life over the past two decades, and several review articles have commented on those so far available. Their use in assessing the outcome of health care interventions has become popular. As we have seen in Chapter 2, recent studies have reported on the quality of life of men with mild to moderate hypertension undergoing antihypertensive therapy, of women with advanced breast cancer undergoing chemotherapy, and of cancer patients in hospice programs.

Although a variety of studies purport to assess quality of life, there is remarkably little agreement about the underlying concepts or theoretical framework that the measures represent. These measures may include clinical symptoms (for example, pain, nausea, vomiting), functional disability (Katz Activities of Daily Living), health status measures (RAND health status measures, Sickness Impact Profile), and measures of life satisfaction and psychological well-being.

The World Health Organization (WHO) has defined health as a "state of complete physical, mental, and social well-being and not merely the absence of disease or infirmity." Ware (1987) argues that five health concepts are inherent in this definition: physical health, mental health, social functioning, role functioning, and general well-being. He takes a conservative approach to the study of quality of life in the health sciences. Because the goal of health care is to maximize the health component of the quality of life, he suggests that the measures be restricted to assessing health status.

Spitzer (1987) includes the burden of symptoms in his operational definition of health. He would restrict the assessment of the attributes of health to those who are definitely sick. He sees little point in extending the studies of quality of life in health care to the ostensibly healthy, but few writers in the field agree with this point of view.

Wenger et al. (1984), McDowell and Newell (1987), and Kane and Kane (1981) offer systematic reviews of a number of measures used in quality-of-life studies, including functional disability indices, health status scales, and measures of life satisfaction. In their reviews, these authors discuss the reliability and validity of a number of the measures and their uses in health care studies. We list the instruments they treat in the section entitled "Three Sources of Descriptive Information for Quality-of-Life Measures." This chapter focuses on measures developed specifically to assess quality of life.

ISSUES IN SELECTING QUALITY-OF-LIFE MEASURES

To choose measures for assessing quality of life, researchers need to address seven issues, briefly reviewed below.

Disease-Specific Versus Global Assessments

Measures may focus on the symptoms, complaints, disabilities, and disruptions in life that are specific to the clinical condition under study. Indeed, the disease-specific approach has been advocated in the study of arthritis, heart disease, and the evaluation of chemotherapy.

Alternatively, one can assess the quality of life resulting from the overall consequences of disease and management on the functional capacities and patients' perception of well-being. The more global measures cover a number of dimensions within a summary score. For example, the Quality of Life Index developed by Spitzer et al. (1981) includes one item for each of the following dimensions: activities of daily living, principal activities, health, outlook, and support. Similarly, measures of life satisfaction and general well-being are global in perspective.

Other measures, such as the linear analogue self-assessment scales developed by Priestman and Baum (1976) or the Breast Cancer Questionnaire (Levine et al. 1988), are designed so that patients may repeatedly assess their symptoms and report their physical and emotional responses to adjuvant chemotherapy. The resulting scores show the patients' immediate and specific responses to disease and treatment.

Clinical Endpoints Versus Long-Term Outcomes

Fletcher et al. (1988) state that the clinical endpoints commonly used for assessing prognoses include evidence of improvement following intervention, remission of disease, and recurrence. Clinical endpoints traditionally focus on sets of outcomes that are assessed near the time of diagnosis and treatment. Long-range outcomes can be viewed as those that are important to patients as they live with their resulting states of health.

Patient Ratings Versus Proxy Assessments

Investigators generally prefer that patients rate their own quality of life. Proxy assessments are important when patients are unable to respond. In these circumstances, researchers may use quality-of-life measures completed by other persons such as a responsible clinician, spouse, close friend, or relative of the patient.

Objective Versus Subjective Measures

Objective measures are based on variables that can be observed and recorded by various testing procedures and assessors. Measures of disease activity, remission of symptoms, presence of side effects, changes in functional capacity, ability to carry out usual activities, and family and social activities are phenomena that can be observed and recorded. These variables are important determinants of quality of life, and agreement can be reached about changes in status that have occurred.

Subjective measures provide opportunities for individuals to express their thoughts, knowledge, attitudes, moods, and feelings. Subjective phenomena may be related to particular diseases or types of therapy, or they may be more global.

Although researchers and policymakers tend to make much of the distinction between objective and subjective measures, both are probably necessary when assessing quality of life, and both require investigations into their reliability and validity. It is perhaps surprising that the objective measures often are not as well standardized as the subjective measures; objectivity does not automatically mean that measures are reliable and valid.

Cognitive Functioning

Researchers commonly exclude cognitive functioning from consideration in studies of quality of life. Except for diseases and therapies that obviously diminish mental capacity, investigators usually assume that the cognitive abilities of individuals are unaffected by episodes of illness and care. One may test this assumption by including tests of cognitive functioning, as did Croog et al. (1986) in their study of antihypertensive medications.

Ratings and Utilities

As Schuessler and Fisher (1985) indicate, quality-of-life measures provide ratings or rankings of health and life. Some assessments attempt to move from states of health to judgments of the worth or value of life with a given state of health. Investigators, working with concepts and methods developed in economics, are designing measures of the utilities of health states, with the typical scores ranging from 0 for "Death" to 1 for "Normal Health." By multiplying the utility values by the number of years individuals live with a given health state, survival time can be expressed in Quality Adjusted Life Years (QALY). Health economists have used this approach to compare technologies in terms of costs per QALY gained. Not everyone agrees with such an approach, because it tends to diminish the value of a good, but troubled, life.

Utility measures move the measurement of quality of life from rankings to judgments of worth and value. This extension of the field of study is controversial; most particularly, the role of utility analysis in quality-of-life research is hotly contested.

Timing of the Assessments

Measures such as the linear analogue self-assessment scales, the Functional Living Index — Cancer, and the Breast Cancer Questionnaire are designed for repeated use before, during, and immediately after treatment. The purpose of the repeated measures is to assess patients' short-term responses during the course of therapy.

Global assessment measures, such as the Spitzer Quality of Life Index, are designed to reflect the quality of life following the impact of disease and management or to reflect global changes in assessments over a long period of time. Investigators have used the Spitzer Quality of Life Index for repeated assessments during the course of therapy (Coates et al. 1987, Levine et al. 1988), but the scores tend to be less responsive to short-term clinical changes than the disease-specific measures.

The basic issue is the use of quality-of-life measures to assess short-term against long-term responses to therapy. For example, Levine et al. (1988) stopped taking assessments when patients withdrew from treatment or relapsed. Conversely, Chubon (1987) used the Life Situation Survey to compare the quality of life of patients in chronic care and rehabilitation programs with those of healthy subjects.

There is a problem with repeated self-assessment during the course of therapy. Investigators have found it difficult to maintain high self-assessment completion rates over several weeks (Finkelstein et al. 1988, Raghavan et al. 1988) and were not able to use the assessments because of missing values. Levine et al. (1988) minimized the problem by having nurses interview the patients during clinic visits; this procedure, however, added considerably to the time and costs of the study. If these measures are to be used repeatedly, the time and costs of maintaining high response rates over multiple assessments must be considered.

Summary

Some quality-of-life studies maintain one perspective or point of view. Yet it is becoming increasingly common for researchers to employ a mix of perspectives and methods in assessing quality of life. We have reviewed what is known about the conceptual framework, reliability, validity, and uses of specific measures. In any study, several tools may be combined to provide information on various perspectives: subjective and objective, disease-specific and global, clinical endpoints and long-term outcomes, and so on. No attempt will be made to sort out the combinations of approaches researchers have employed. Examples of multiple approaches to assessing quality of life are given in Chapter 2.

STRATEGIES USED TO ASSESS INSTRUMENTS

A bewildering array of terms labels the properties of measures, and researchers in the health sciences frequently employ strategies for developing and testing measures that differ from those used in the social sciences. To standardize our work, we developed the Review Form for Quality-of-Life Measures. We used the Review Form to gather bibliographic information, the stated purpose of the measure, its underlying conceptual framework, and a description of its content and format. As part of this review, we have tried to use terms that are consistent with those compiled in the *Dictionary of Epidemiology* (Last 1988) by the International Epidemiology Association and that are used by writers in epidemiology (Feinstein 1987, McDowell and Newell 1987) and the social sciences (Bohrnstedt 1981, Kerlinger 1986, Nunnally 1978). This section briefly reviews some statistical and other expressions.

Reliability

Two basic strategies can be used to establish the reliability of a measure. For those based on subjective ratings of attitudes, perceptions, and sense of well-being, investigators may assess the reliability by examining the consistency of patterns of response across the items. The coefficient alpha (Cronbach 1951) measures the internal consistency of the response, based on the average correlation among the items and the number of items in the instrument. The coefficient assumes that the correlations in the matrix are all positive, because they represent the same dimension. Values of Cronbach's alpha range from 0 to 1.

If Cronbach's alpha is high (for example, 0.80 or higher), the responses are consistent, and the sum of the item responses yields a score for the underlying dimensions that the item represents. Stated another way, if the items are adequately sampled from the domain of quality of life, the sum of the responses should give a better indication of the quality of life of the individual than the response to any one item. A low coefficient alpha would indicate that the items did not come from the same conceptual domain or that the noise in the items was substantial.

The items can be divided and placed on alternate forms of the measure; the equivalence of the alternate forms can be tested by comparing the alphas. Alternatively, the items on one form can be split into two groups, and coefficients can be computed for each half and compared. Comparable coefficients confirm the consistency of the responses.

The scores for the split forms can also be correlated to see how they correspond. The Spearman-Brown formula uses this correlation to estimate the reliability of a scale containing all items after adjusting for the presence of twice as many items on the composite scale as in each of the two groups (Zeller and Carmines 1980).

Researchers may decide to create a multidimensional measure of quality of life and then select items that represent the dimensions of interest. For example, quality-of-life measures may have items related to conditions specific to disease and management (for example, nausea and vomiting in response to chemotherapy for cancer), and there may be additional items related to physical functioning, and social and psychological well-being.

Factor analysis statistically defines a small number of factors or underlying dimensions that account for a high proportion of the common variance of the items. Exploratory factor analysis is used to identify and discard items that are not correlated with the factors of interest. Alternatively, an investigator may use factor analysis to confirm that items selected to represent a single dimension of quality of life (for example, physical functioning) principally load onto that factor and correlate weakly with other factors. The factor represents a single dominant dimension or variable when the factor loadings for the items are relatively high — 0.60 or higher—and the common variance and the factor loadings cannot be increased by subdividing the items onto additional factors. Factors are not considered stable unless the results can be replicated in a number of samples and study settings. Once a factor is defined as representing a single variable or dimension, the responses for the items on each factor are summed to create the factor score.

For a measure with a fairly large number of items and a high coefficient alpha, one can use factor analysis to define two or more factors underlying the responses. A measure that is internally consistent may still not represent a single dimension. Factor analysis is used to define the underlying dimensions, and the coefficient alpha may then be used to assess the strength of the consistency of the items on the separate factors.

The stability of a scale or factor score is assessed by correlating the scores of subjects with the scores obtained in testing at another time. As Bohrnstedt (1981) has noted, the test-retest coefficient can be influenced by true changes in scores. The interpretation of the coefficient of stability is not always straightforward.

If the variables being considered are sufficiently objective to be evaluated by persons other than the patients, it is possible to compare raters' scores. For example, the Quality of Life Index is designed to be completed by the health professional responsible for the care of the patient and significant others as well as by patients themselves. Interrater agreement indicates the reliability of the scores by different raters on a single occasion, and intrarater agreement is the reliability of the scores by the same rater over repeated testings.

If the measure is categorical, Cohen's kappa (Fleiss 1981) is most frequently used to assess the level of agreement beyond that expected by chance. For rankings of ordinal measures, Spearman's rho and Kendall's tau may be used as measures of agreement in addition to kappa. Pearson's product moment correlation is commonly used for comparing quantitative scores of raters.

The preferred measure of agreement is the intraclass correlation coefficient. It is particularly useful when there are three or more ratings. It compares the variance between subjects, the variance between raters, and the variance between times with the error variance. The intraclass correlation is reliable if most of the variance in the model is accounted for by the variance between subjects and if the variances by raters and by time are minimal (Fleiss 1986). The measure rests on the analysis of variance and can be used with ordinal as well as interval data. An intraclass correlation coefficient of, for example, 0.80 or higher indicates that the measure is highly reliable.

Scaling refers to the rules for assigning numbers to responses. The scaling determines whether the measure is a nominal, ordinal, interval, or ratio variable.

Validity

A first step in assessing the validity of a measure is to determine if the content of the items represents the domain or dimension of interest. Face validity is sometimes used to refer to the intuitive appeal of the items; content validity is reserved for the judgments of experts or specialists.

When there exists a variable external to the measure against which the scores can be checked, that variable can be used as a criterion to judge the measures. For example, the quality-of-life scores should differentiate patients dying of cancer, patients in intensive care, outpatients with chronic diseases, and healthy individuals, even though there may be substantial overlaps in the distributions of scores.

Concurrent criterion validity refers to the ability of a measure to differentiate between groups at the time the measure is applied. Predictive criterion validity refers to the ability to use these scores to predict future health-related events and states.

Quality-of-life measures can be compared with other measures as well. Concepts derived from theory and operationalized into reliable and valid measures are referred to as constructs. The measures under study can be tested against the constructs to determine if the observed relationships are as hypothesized. For example, quality of life should be negatively related to measures of pain, anxiety, and depression. Similarly, a measure of quality of life should be positively related to life satisfaction and general well-being.

To judge the sensitivity or responsiveness of a measure, the investigator should have a sense of how much change in a patient's clinical or functional status would produce a change in their quality-of-life score. Significant clinical changes in the individual may not parallel changes in quality-of-life scores. Alternatively, a relatively small change in clinical levels may result in marked changes in a patient's sense of psychological well-being.

Finally, the practicality of a measure refers to the ease and convenience of administration and interpretation. Practicality is particularly important if a measure is to be used repeatedly.

A REVIEW OF SELECTED MEASURES FOR ASSESSING QUALITY OF LIFE

We reviewed 10 measures for rating quality of life using the Review Form for Quality-of-Life Measures. The section entitled "Ten Review Forms for Quality-of-Life Measures" presents the completed forms, and Table 6-1 (see page 76, this volume) provides a summary.

The Quality of Life Index (QLI), developed by Spitzer et al. (1981), has been tested in a variety of settings. It is used to assess the physical, psychological, and social functioning of patients. The QLI yields a score that ranges from a high of 10 to a low of 0. Alternative forms for completion by the patient, the physician or other health professional, relative, or significant other were developed to determine whether comparable ratings could be obtained from several sources. The reliability and validity of the QLI have been demonstrated in a series of studies in Australia, Canada, and the United States with a variety of patients.

Chubon (1987), Padilla et al. (1983), and Ferrans and Powers (1985) developed global measures of quality of life to be completed by patients. Chubon's Life Situation Survey assesses quality of life beyond disease-specific conditions and functional limitations, comparing the responses of patients in chronic care and rehabilitation programs with those of healthy subjects. Chubon tested his instrument with prison inmates, hospital patients, mentally retarded adults, spinal injury patients, and university students. Although the samples have been relatively small, the instrument appeared to work well with all groups, and the differences in mean scores were as predicted. Chubon also found positive changes in the mean scores of patients who completed a program for chronic back pain.

Padilla's Quality of Life Index focused on physical conditions, activities, and attitudes of the patients. We found no reports of the measures other than the articles published by the developers of the instruments. Padilla originally developed her measure while working with cancer patients. She adapted the measure for use with colostomy patients, adding a number of disease-specific items. Although the measure was designed to be global, we found no use of the adapted measure across conditions.

Ferrans' Quality of Life Index focused on the satisfaction of needs; this measure is broader in scope. It taps life satisfaction in areas outside the immediate reach of health care (for example, marriage, education, occupation, future retirement), in addition to items related directly to health. By 1988, results had been reported for healthy graduate students and dialysis patients.

Karnofsky and Burchemal (1949) were among the first to develop a measure to assess the ability of cancer patients to perform daily activities. Their measure has been studied extensively and is widely used, although it has been criticized both conceptually and for its measurement properties. The consensus seems to be that it continues to be a useful tool for physicians to use in rating the impact of cancer and cancer treatment on patients' ability to lead normal lives.

The Functional Living Index — Cancer (FLIC) is one of the newer instruments. The FLIC contains 22 items pertaining to symptoms and complaints related to cancer treatment, as well as the impact of disease and management on physical, psychological, and social functioning. The items were tested on 837 patients in Winnipeg and Edmonton, Canada. When the data were factor analyzed, Schipper et al. (1984) found that the mean factor scores for four patient groups decreased with the extent of disease. The investigators have completed some construct validation exercises. The FLIC is designed to be completed daily by patients. The responsiveness of the scores to changes over time has yet to be established.

Selby et al. (1984) have taken another approach to the development of an instrument for cancer patients. They took 18 items from the Sickness Impact Profile and added 12 items based on clinical experience, along with 2 statements for a global rating of quality of life and life satisfaction. The resulting questionnaire is designed to be completed by either physicians or patients. Factor analysis has been used to define the dimensions the items represent. The changes in scores reflect response to chemotherapy. We found no reports of uses of the instrument by investigators other than Selby and his colleagues.

TABLE 6-1 A Summary of Health-Related Quality-of-Life Measures

Measure	Quality of Life Index	Life Situation Survey	Quality of Life Index
First author	Spitzer	Chubon	Padilla
Assessment	Global	Global	Disease-specific
Rater	Patient, clinician, significant other	Subject	Patient
Subjects	Healthy, cancer patients, seriously ill, chronically ill, terminally ill	Students, inmates, patients (ESRD,[a] back, spinal injury, mentally retarded)	Patients (cancer, chemotherapy or radiotherapy, diabetics, healthy)
Dimensions	Principal activity, activities of daily living, health, social support, outlook on life	Life quality	Physical condition, daily activities, personal attitudes
Reliability			
Internal consistency	**	**	*
Rater	**	—	—
Stability	**	*	*
Validity			
Content	**	*	*
Criterion			
Concurrent	**	**	*
Predictive	*	*	—
Construct	**	—	*
Responsiveness	*	—	—
Applications by others	**	—	—

Measure	Quality of Life Index	Quality of Life Index	Karnofsky Index of Performance Status	Functional Living Index — Cancer
First author	Padilla	Ferrans	Karnofsky	Schipper
Assessment	Disease-specific	Global	Cancer-specific	Cancer-specific
Rater	Patient	Subject	Physician	Patient
Subjects	Colostomy patients	Healthy persons, dialysis patients	Patients	Patients
Dimensions	Psychological and physical well-being, body image, diagnosis/treatment, surgical and nutritional response, social concerns	Health care, physical functioning, marriage, family, friends, stress, occupation, education, leisure, retirement, peace of mind, faith, life goals, appearance, happiness, satisfaction	Physical status, physical activities	Symptoms, sociability, daily living, satisfaction
Reliability				
Internal consistency	*	*	—	**
Rater	—	—	*	—
Stability	—	*	*	*
Validity				
Content	*	*	*	**
Criterion				
Concurrent	—	—	*	*
Predictive	—	—	*	—
Construct	*	*	**	*
Responsiveness	—	—	*	—
Applications by others	—	—	**	—

Measure	Study (*unnamed*)	Linear Analogue Self-Assessment Scale	Breast Cancer Questionnaire
First author	Selby	Priestman	Levine
Assessment	Cancer-specific	Disease-specific	Cancer-specific
Rater	Patient, physician	Patient	Interviewer
Subjects	Cancer patients	Patients (cancers of breast, lung, bladder)	Breast cancer patients
Dimensions	12 categories of SIP, clinical problems	Symptoms, side effects, anxiety, depression, personal relations, physical performance	Consequences of hair loss, emotional dysfunction, physical symptoms, trouble with treatment, fatigue, nausea, positive well-being
Reliability			
Internal consistency	*	—	—
Rater	*	—	—
Stability	*	*	*
Validity			
Content	*	—	**
Criterion			
Concurrent	—	*	—
Predictive	—	*	*
Construct	*	*	*
Responsiveness	*	*	*
Applications by others	*	*	—

NOTE: Symbols are as follows: —, not assessed; *, assessed; **, strong feature.
[a] End-stage renal disease.

We found considerable discussion of linear analogue self-assessment (LASA) or visual analogue scales (VAS) for rating quality of life. These scales are typically 10 centimeters long with the low or poor end of the scale anchored at 0 and the upper end anchored at 100. In response to a cue word or phrase, patients mark their self-assessments on the line. The point marked to the nearest millimeter produces the score. Priestman and Baum (1976) were among the first to use this technique for quality-of-life assessments of cancer patients. In a number of studies these and other investigators have used items related to symptoms and side effects, anxiety and depression, personal relations, and functioning, but the actual cues have varied from study to study.

The scores from repeated testing over the course of treatment for advanced cancer have been reported for individual items, but we found no reports of the formal psychometric properties in the measure. A minority of eligible subjects participated in the repeated use of the form, but the loss to follow-up is not explained. The use of the LASA needs to be standardized so that measurement properties of the resulting scales can be formally tested.

Three trends can be observed in the development of quality-of-life measures. First, although investigators have focused on the clinical relevance of the measures, minimal attention has been paid to the conceptual underpinnings of quality of life or the theoretical bases for the particular measures. Second, most researchers develop and modify the measures without formally testing the reliability, validity, and responsiveness of the resulting scores. Third, the various measures have been developed in isolation from each other, and attempts to compare and contrast the various measures of quality of life are rare.

A REVIEW OF UTILITY ASSESSMENTS IN QUALITY OF LIFE

The utility assessment of health states and quality of life has arisen from a theoretical perspective and methodology that are distinct from those employed by behavioral and clinical scientists. Utility assessment has two components, the judgment of the value or worth of life at a given point in time and the quantity or years of life spent in various health states.

The utility value assigned to a health state generally ranges from 0, the value ascribed to death, to 1, the value ascribed to the reference state of a healthy life. By multiplying a utility value for a health state by the number of years of duration of the expected health state, the resulting product is the Quality Adjusted Life Years (QALY). Health economists posit that health care programs should be evaluated by comparing the relative costs of the programs with the QALYs produced.

The general approach for assessing utility values is based on modern utility theory, advanced by von Neumann and Morgenstern (1953). The theory describes a method for decisionmaking under conditions of uncertainty based on a set of axioms of rational behavior. Holloway (1979) has summarized the wide uses of this model for decisionmaking. Drummond et al. (1986), Torrance (1986, 1987), and Weinstein (1983) have written reviews and summaries of the utility analysis of health care programs. Smith (1988) has presented a number of papers with applications of utility analysis. The reader may wish to refer to these sources for detailed discussions of the theory and methods of utility analysis.

The major groups of researchers responsible for applying utility theory to the health field include the late James Bush, Robert Kaplan, and their colleagues at the University of California at San Diego; Rachel Rosser and her colleagues at Charing Cross Hospital in London; George Torrance and his colleagues at McMaster University in Hamilton, Ontario; and Milton Weinstein and his colleagues at Harvard University. Torrance (1986, 1987) and Kaplan and his associates (Kaplan et al. 1984, Anderson et al. 1988) have published information on the reliability and validity of their methods, and we review their works briefly.

The description of the health state is the first step in deriving utility values. Torrance et al. (1982) have identified six attributes that should be included in a description of health state: physical function, emotional function, sensory function, cognitive function, self-care, and pain. The description would indicate the level of functioning on each of the attributes associated with a particular health state. The descriptions can be presented in narrative paragraphs, videotapes of patients, or in other forms.

The descriptions are presented to patients with the given health states, their close relatives or friends, or health care professionals for judgments of the utility values to be assigned to the states. The utility values may be rated on a visual analogue scale ranging from 0 to 100, with 0 indicating the worse possible health state (death) and 100 the best possible health state. This method is referred to as a rating scale.

The standard gamble technique was the original method for deriving utility values. It sits directly on the axioms of utility theory. The subject uses the standard gamble to choose between two alternatives to treatment. The outcome of an intervention (new procedure) may be a good outcome with a given probability (for example, 80 percent chance of restoration to normal health) or a worse outcome with a given probability (such as a 20 percent chance of permanent disability or death). The second intervention (for example, another treatment or no treatment at all) is presented with a certain (100 percent sure) outcome of intermediate desirability relative to the good and bad outcomes associated with the first intervention. The probabilities associated with the new intervention (p for a good outcome, $1 - p$ for a bad outcome) are varied until the subject perceives no real difference between the interventions, and the utility value is then calculated for the various health states of the second intervention. Torrance (1986) reported that the standard gamble method can be used to measure utilities for chronic health states preferred to death, chronic states considered worse than death, and temporary health states.

Torrance et al. (1972) developed the time trade-off method for use in health care evaluations, and they claim it is simpler to use than the standard gamble approach. The subject considers a health state associated with a problem that is to last for a fixed period of time as opposed to a shorter period of healthy life. The subject is asked to "trade off" the time in a compromised health state with a lesser time in a healthier state. The time in the healthy state is varied until the point of indifference is found, and the utility value is calculated accordingly.

With six key attributes and multiple levels on each attribute, a large number of unique health states would have to be defined to describe all possible combinations of attributes. Torrance et al. (1982) have used multiple attribute theory to reduce the number of measurements required to obtain the utility values for all combinations of attribute levels.

Torrance (1987) presented a summary of the reliability ratings and tests of validity of the utility values from the rating, standard gamble, and time trade-off methods. The interrater and test-retest reliabilities range from 0.63 to 0.88. The results of the rating scales and time trade-off methods have been validated through comparisons with the standard gamble approach. (Torrance refers to this as criterion validity for the standard gamble method because it is derived directly from the axioms of utility theory. We refer to this as construct validity because the standard gamble method is a scientific construct for inferring preferences in decisionmaking.) Churchill and his associates (1987) compared time trade-off utilities of end-stage renal disease patients with the ratings of physicians on the Quality of Life Index and found them to be congruent. That is, they demonstrated construct validity.

The methods are time consuming, demanding of the subjects, and costly to apply. The McMaster group has refined the methods and simplified the tasks. They have achieved participation and task completion rates of at least 85 percent.

The San Diego group has taken a different approach to assessing utility values (Kaplan et al. 1984, Kaplan and Bush 1982). Their first step was to categorize individuals in given health states with respect to levels of mobility, physical activity, and social activity. The second step was to classify the same individuals by the symptoms and health problems that they have on a given day. Four hundred case descriptions were written to encompass the combinations of functional levels and symptoms or problems.

Random samples of individuals in a community gave preference ratings to the descriptions on a continuum ranging from 0 for death to 1 for completely well. A model for preference structure assigned weights to each level of functioning and symptoms/problem complex. Quality of Well-Being scores are derived by applying the weights for functional levels and symptoms/problems to health states of interest, and the Quality of Well-Being (QWB) scores are the utility values for those states.

Anderson et al. (1988) compared the reliability of the QWB scores in general household samples and a clinical outcome study of burn patients. In initial interviews, the subjects completed self-administered forms and personal interviews. In a follow-up survey they repeated the process. They used internal consistency analysis to detect discrepancies in responses and reported that 50 percent of the discrepancies were the result of correctable errors. They concluded that personal interviews are required for the reliable use of the QWB.

We found no published reports that compare the utility values derived by the standard gamble, time trade-off, and rating scale methods outlined by Torrance with the QWB utility values developed by the San Diego group.

Several questions and criticisms have been directed toward the use of utility values and QALYs in quality-of-life assessments. Some experts debate whether the utility values should be obtained from the public at large, the providers, or the patients themselves. Others argue that the utility assessments are incomplete unless they include the perspectives of the family members whose lives are directly affected by the health status and quality of life of the patients. If the patient is unable to form a judgment, should the next of kin or some close friend be asked to make a decision about the perceived utility of the patient's health status and prognosis?

Patients' assessments of the utility of health states change as their health does. For this reason, utility values may not be stable over long periods of time. Furthermore, projections about morbidity, disability, and mortality frequently depend on expert opinion in the absence of sound epidemiological data on the natural history of disease and the impact of interventions. Consequently, assumptions about life expectancy may be only crude estimates of actual experience.

Experts do not agree on the key attributes to be included. Torrance advocates the inclusion of physical, emotional, sensory, cognitive, and self-care functioning, in addition to pain, but he excludes social functioning. In actual use the descriptions used in the standard gamble and time trade-off methods vary according to the disease or technology being evaluated. The QWB is narrow in focus because it encompasses only mobility, physical activity, social activity, and symptoms.

Lastly, although individuals may understand and agree with the ratings for the levels of functioning for a set of attributes, they agree less when the issue is whether a derived utility value accurately reflects the worth of human life. The public has even more skepticism about multiplying the life expectancy times the utility values to obtain a "quality-adjusted life year." In summary, utility assessments of quality of life can at best be described as technology with promise and potential, but not as one accepted by the public.

THREE SOURCES OF DESCRIPTIVE INFORMATION FOR QUALITY-OF-LIFE MEASURES

The editors and the authors of this chapter refer readers to three books for reviews of more extensively studied and firmly established quality-of-life measures. The first, *Assessment of Quality of Life in Clinical Trials of Cardiovascular Therapies,* reviews six quality-of-life instruments and provides information on their content, administration, development, validity, reliability, generalizability, applications, and major strengths and limitations. The book lists references for these instruments, contains reproductions of many of them, and compares and contrasts them. The citation for the book and the names of instruments included are:

Wenger, N.K., Mattson, M.E., Furberg, C.D., and Elinson, J., eds. Assessment of Quality of Life in Clinical Trials of Cardiovascular Therapies. New York, Le Jacq Publishing, Inc., 1984

- Sickness Impact Profile (SIP)
- Quality of Well-Being (QWB) Scale
- Psychological General Well-Being (PGWB) Index
- McMaster Health Index Questionnaire (MHIQ)

- Nottingham Health Profile (NHP)
- General Health Rating Index (GHRI)

The second book is entitled *Measuring Health: A Guide to Rating Scales and Questionnaires*. It reviews measures by name, developers, purpose, conceptual basis, and description. It offers information on reliability and validity, alternative forms of each instrument (if any), references, commentaries on strengths and limitations, the addresses of the original test developers, and complete or partial reproductions of the instruments. Each review has been checked for accuracy and completeness by the instrument developers.

This book features a "consumer's guide" to the various instruments, which provides information on numerical characteristics of the scale, length, applications, method of administration, a rating of how widely each instrument is used, and a rating of reliability and validity. The citation for the book and the names of instruments listed are:

McDowell, I., and Newell, C. Measuring Health: A Guide to Rating Scales and Questionnaires. New York, Oxford University Press, Inc., 1987.

Activities of Daily Living (ADL) Scales

- The PULSES Profile (Physical condition, Upper limb functions, Lower limb functions, Sensory components, Excretory functions, mental and emotional Status)
- The Barthel Index
- The Index of Independence in Activities of Daily Living, or Index of ADL
- The Kenney Self-Care Evaluation
- The Physical Self-Maintenance Scale
- The Functional Status Rating System

Instrumental Activities of Daily Living (IADL) Scales

- A Rapid Disability Rating Scale
- The Functional Status Index
- The Patient Evaluation Conference System
- The Functional Activities Questionnaire
- The Lambeth Disability Screening Questionnaire
- The Disability and Impairment Interview Schedule

Psychological Indices

- The Health Opinion Survey
- The 22 Item Screening Score of Psychiatric Symptoms

- The Affect Balance Scale
- The General Well-Being Schedule
- The Mental Health Inventory
- The General Health Questionnaire

Social Health Indices

- The Social Relationship Scale
- The Social Support Questionnaire
- The Social Maladjustment Schedule
- The Katz Adjustment Scales
- The Social Health Battery
- The Social Dysfunction Rating Scale
- The Social Functioning Schedule
- The Interview Schedule for Social Interaction
- The Structured and Scaled Interview to Assess Maladjustment
- The Social Adjustment Scale

Quality-of-Life and Life Satisfaction Indices

- The Quality of Life Index
- Four Single-Item Indicators of Well-Being
- The Life Satisfaction Index
- The Philadelphia Geriatric Center Morale Scale

Pain Measurements

- Visual Analogue Pain Rating Scales
- The Oswestry Low Back Pain Disability Questionnaire
- The McGill Pain Questionnaire
- The Self-Rating Pain and Distress Scale
- The Illness Behavior Questionnaire
- The Pain Perception Profile

General Health Measurements

- The Arthritis Impact Measurement Scale
- The Physical and Mental Impairment-of-Function Evaluation
- The Functional Assessment Inventory
- The Nottingham Health Profile
- The Sickness Impact Profile
- The Multilevel Assessment Instrument
- The Older Americans Resources and Services (OARS) Multidimensional Functional Assessment Questionnaire
- The Comprehensive Assessment and Referral Evaluation
- The Quality of Well-Being Scale

The third book, *Assessing the Elderly: A Practical Guide to Measurement*, contains reviews of instruments in four major areas of measurement important to long-term care (LTC) providers: physical functioning, mental functioning, social functioning, and multidimensional or composite measures. It outlines methods of administration, reliability and validity; types of scales used; the strengths and limitations of the measures; and their similarities and differences and lists their items and characteristics according to function and purpose. It also offers practical suggestions for their use. The authors also cite unpublished instruments — "perhaps circulated at professional meetings"—that may be of interest to researchers developing or modifying instruments. The book citation and a partial list of instruments are as follows:

Kane, R.A., and Kane, R.L. Assessing the Elderly: A Practical Guide to Measurement. Lexington, Massachusetts, D.C. Heath and Company, 1981.

Measures of Physical Functioning
Measures of Physical Health

- Cornell Medical Index
- Cumulative Illness Rating Scale
- Health Index
- Patient Appraisal and Care Evaluation (PACE) II: Medical Data
- Patient Classification for Long-Term Care (LTC): Impairments and Medical Status
- Older Americans Resources and Services (OARS): Physical Health

Measures of Ability to Perform Activities of Daily Living (ADL) or Physical Functioning

- PULSES Profile
- Index of ADL
- Kenney Self-Care Evaluation
- Barthel Index Rapid Disability Rating Scale (RDRS)
- Barthel Self-Care Ratings
- Granger Range of Motion Scale
- Kenney Self-Care Evaluation
- PACE II: Physical Function
- OARS: Physical ADL
- Functional Health Status of the Institutionalized Elderly ADL-A

Measures of Ability to Perform Instrumental Activities of Daily Living (IADL)

- Functional Health Status
- PGC Instrumental Activities of Daily Living
- Instrumental Role Maintenance Scale
- PACE II: IADLs
- OARS: Instrumental ADL
- Functioning for Independent Living
- Performance Activities of Daily Living (PADL)
- Pilot Geriatric Arthritis Project Functional Status Measure (PGAP)

Measures of Mental Functioning
Measures of Cognitive Functioning

- Vigor, Intactness, Relationships, and Orientation (VIRO) Orientation Scale
- Mental Status Questionnaire (MSQ)
- Short Portable Mental Status Questionnaire (SPMSQ) from OARS
- Philadelphia Geriatric Center (PGC) Mental Status Questionnaire
- PGC Extended Mental Status Questionnaire
- Memory and Information Test (MIT)
- Dementia Rating Scale (DRS)
- Extended Scale for Dementia
- Face-Hands Test
- Visual Counting Test
- Set Test
- Misplaced Objects Test
- Wechsler Adult Intelligence Scale (WAIS) Short Form
- Wechsler Memory Test
- Quick Test (QT)
- Mini-Mental State Examination
- Geriatric Interpersonal Evaluation Scale (GIES)

Measures of Affective Functioning

- Zung Self-Rating Depression Scale (SDS)
- Beck Depression Index
- Hopkins Symptom Checklist
- Affect-Balance Scale

Measures of General Mental Health

- OARS Mental Health Screening

- Screening Score
- Emotional Problems Questionnaire
- Savage-Britten Index
- Sandoz Clinical Assessment — Geriatrics
- London (Ontario) Psychogeriatric Rating Scale (LPRS)
- Gerontological Apperception Test (GAT)
- Senior Apperception Test (SAT)
- Geriatric Mental State Examination
- Psychological Well-Being Interview
- Nurses Observation Scale for Impatient Evaluation (NOSIE)

Measures of Social Functioning
Measures of Social Interactions and Resources

- Network Analysis Profile
- Social Networks Assessment Questionnaire
- Role Activity Scales
- Mutual Support Index
- Family Structure and Contact Battery (1968)
- Exchanges Between the Generations Index
- Family Structure and Contact Battery (1972)
- Exchanges of Support and Assistance Index
- Hebrew Rehabilitation Center for the Aged (HRCA) Social Interaction Inventory
- Bennett Social Isolation Scales
- Family Adaptation, Partnership, Growth, Affection, Resolve (APGAR)
- OARS Social Resources Scale
- Social Dysfunction Rating Scale
- Social Behavior Assessment
- HRCA Reduced Activities Inventory
- Activity Scale
- Unusual Day
- Future Activity Scores

Measures of Subjective Well-Being and Coping

- Cavan Attitude Inventory
- Kutner Morale Scale
- Life Satisfaction Index
- Oberleder Attitude Scale
- Contentment Scale
- Tri-Scales

- PGC Morale Scale
- Geriatric Coping Schedule
- Mode of Adaptations Patterns Scale
- Geriatric Scale of Recent Life Events

Measures of Person-Environment Fit

- Importance, Locus, and Range of Activities Check-list
- Locus of Desired Control
- Perceived Environmental Constraint Index
- Satisfaction with Nursing Home Scale
- Home for the Aged Description Questionnaire
- Ward Atmosphere Scale
- Community-Oriented Programs Environment Scale (COPES)
- Sheltered Care Environment
- Person-Environment Fit
- Person-Environment Fit Scale

Multidimensional Measures

- Sickness Impact Profile (SIP)
- Older Americans Research and Service (OARS) Center Instrument
- Comprehensive Assessment and Referral Evaluation (CARE)
- Patient Appraisal and Care Evaluation (PACE)
- Stockton Geriatric Rating Scale
- Plutchik Geriatric Rating Scale
- Parachek Geriatric Rating Scale
- Physical and Mental Impairment-of-Function Evaluation Scale (PAMIE)

We also refer readers to the Clearinghouse on Health Indexes of the National Center for Health Statistics of the U.S. Department of Health and Human Services. The Clearinghouse publishes a quarterly *Bibliography on Health Indexes* (editor, P. Erickson) that provides information on the reliability, validity, and sensitivity of various measures of health status.

TEN REVIEW FORMS FOR QUALITY-OF-LIFE MEASURES

The review forms give, where available, the name of the measure, the author(s), primary reference(s), purpose, conceptual framework, description, reliability (including internal consistency, equivalence, stability, interrater reliability, scaling, and scalability), validity (content, concurrent, predictive, and construct), sensitivity, practicality, references, and applications (sometimes with descriptions).

1. Review Form for Quality of Life Index and Quality of Life Uniscale

Name of Measure: Quality of Life Index—Spitzer
Quality of Life Uniscale—Spitzer
Authors: Spitzer, W.O., Dobson, A.J., Hall, J., Chesterman, E., Levi, J., Shepherd, R., Battista, R.N., and Catchlove, B.R.

Primary References:

Measuring the quality of life of cancer patients: A concise QL-index for use by physicians. Journal of Chronic Diseases 34(12):585-597, 1981.
Mor, V. Cancer patients quality of life over the disease course: Lessons from the real world. Journal of Chronic Diseases 40(6):535-544, 1987.
Morris, J.N., Suissa, S., Sherwood, S., Wright, S.M., and Greer, D. Last days: A study of the quality of life of terminally ill cancer patients. Journal of Chronic Diseases 39(1):47-62, 1986.

Purpose: The Quality of Life Index (QLI) provides a measure to help physicians assess the relative benefits and risks of treatments for serious illness and of supportive programs such as palliative care or hospice service.

Conceptual Framework: The QLI covers five dimensions: occupational, household, or other principal activities; activities of daily living; health; support of family members or other significant persons; and outlook on life. It was designed to provide a global measure of these dimensions; it was not designed to be a measure of functional health status. The QLI Uniscale is a visual analogue scale on which the subject is asked to provide a global summary rating. The instruments are designed for use by patients, significant others, and attending health professionals.

Reliability:
Internal consistency: 91 subjects in Australia, alpha = 0.76, Brown Cancer and Aging study, alpha = 0.80, Brown Concrete Needs study, alpha = 0.77, National Hospice study, alpha = 0.66.

Interrater: Spearman correlations of physicians' ratings were 0.84 (English) and 0.74 (Francophone). Physician-patient correlations were 0.61 (Australia) and 0.69 (Canada).

Scalability: Possible scores for each dimension are 0 (attribute in activity essentially absent), 1 (attribute or activity partially present), or 2 (attribute or activity fully present, normal). QLI scores range from 0 to 10. Anchoring adjectives are lowest quality and highest quality. The position of the mark on the line may be measured to the nearest millimeter or centimeter.

Validity:
Content: Content validity was based on a review of the literature and on information supplied by content panels of patients with various diseases, their relatives, healthy persons, physicians, other health professionals, and clergy. Items were selected in a three-stage process; the final choices were based on methodological and content criteria.

Concurrent: In Australia, measures showed mean differences between 84 healthy individuals in Sydney, 101 healthy individuals in Hunter Valley, 108 chronically ill patients, 105 cancer patients, and 78 seriously ill patients in hospital. It also differentiated newly diagnosed cancer patients, ($n = 397$), recipients of chemotherapy ($n = 194$), and terminally ill patients in the Brown studies. Scores are related to type of treatment in end-stage renal disease.

Predictive: In the National Hospice Study, QLI scores declined over the last six weeks of the lives of patients.

Construct: The QLI and QLI Uniscale have been related to the Karnofsky Index and measures of pain, depression, and nausea in the Brown studies. They have been compared with Linear Analogue Self-Assessment (LASA) measures in Australian Breast Cancer studies. QLI scores were compared with time trade-off utilities for end-stage renal disease patients by Churchill et al. (1987).

Sensitivity: QLI scores show deterioration over the last few weeks of the lives of patients in a hospice program. It has been used to demonstrate variable response to chemotherapy.

Practicality: The instrument is short, easy to understand, and brief. The scores from 0 to 10 have an intuitive appeal.

References and Applications:

Churchill, D.N., Torrance, G.W., Taylor, D.W., Barnes, C.C., Ludwin, D., Schimizu, A., and Smith, E.K. Measurement of quality of life in end-stage renal disease: The time trade-off approach. Clinical and Investigative Medicine 10(1):14-20, 1987.

Coates, A., Gebski, V., Bishop, J.F., Jeal, P.N., Woods, R.L., Snyder, R., Tattersall, M.H., Byrne, M., Harvey, V., and Gill, G., for the Australian-New Zealand Breast Cancer Trials Group, Clinical Oncology Society of Australia. Improving the quality of life during chemotherapy for advanced breast cancer. A comparison of intermittent and continuous treatment strategies. New England Journal of Medicine 317(24):1490-1495, 1987.

Three hundred and eight patients with advanced breast cancer were randomized to continuous or intermittent chemotherapy. Quality of life was measured with five LASA scores for physical well-being, mood, pain, nausea, vomiting, and appetite; the QLI Uniscale was completed by patients, and the QLI by physicians. All scores showed that patients reported higher quality of life with continuous rather than intermittent therapy. This was consistent with the patients' clinical responses.

Gough, I.R., Furnival, C.M., Schilder, L., and Grove, W. Assessment of the quality of life of patients with advanced cancer. European Journal of Cancer and Clinical Oncology 19(8):1161-1165, 1983.

One hundred patients completed 335 sets of LASA forms that included 21 LASA items; in addition the same 100 patients were rated on the QLI administered by a social worker, the QLI completed by patients, and a single well-being (LASA) item. Investigators found that the highest correlations were between social workers' and patients' responses to the QLI. Single-item well-being was judged to be as useful as the 21-item form.

2. Review Form for Life Situation Survey

Name of Measure: Life Situation Survey
Author: Chubon, R.A.

Primary Reference:

A quality of life rating scale. Evaluation and the Health Professions 10:186-200, 1987.

Purpose: The Life Situation Survey is a subjective instrument that can be used in a variety of populations, including patients in chronic care and rehabilitation programs.

Conceptual Framework: Chubon is critical of quality-of-life measures that are disease-specific or focus on functional limitations. Chubon focuses on the subjective aspect of life quality that may be more critical to understanding the impact of treatment. The Life Situation Survey includes 20 statements; respondents indicate the degree to which they agree or disagree with the statements by checking six-point rating categories. A midpoint, the seventh category, was omitted and reserved for assignment of a score where no response was recorded. Half of the items are positively worded; the other half are negatively worded. Scores range from 20 to 140.

Reliability:

Stability: The test-retest reliability for 23 graduate students over one week was 0.91.

Internal consistency: Cronbach's alpha for a variety of groups ranges from 0.74 to 0.95. The groups include prison inmates, hospital patients, university students, mentally retarded individuals employed in workshops, and spinal cord injury patients in rehabilitation.

Scalability: The scores from the seven response categories are summed over the 20 items.

Validity:

Content: Items were developed by asking 168 persons with a variety of chronic and disabling conditions to indicate difficulties experienced as a result of this condition and actions that could be taken to improve the quality of their lives. The items were sorted into 17 categories through pilot tests. Twenty items for 10 categories were developed for the form.

Concurrent: Chubon (1987) investigated the concurrent validity of the Life Situation Survey using several groups. Chubon found that the means of inmate and patient groups were significantly different from the student group mean. Sample sizes, means, and standard deviations are displayed in Table 6-2.

TABLE 6-2 Sample Sizes, Means, and Standard Deviations for the Life Situation Survey

Feature	Students	Medium Security Inmates	End-Stage Renal Disease Patients	Back Problem Patients	Spinal Injury Patients	Mentally Retarded Individuals
Sample size	50	44	27	22	16	30
Mean	107.3	74.3	83.2	81.1	87.9	102.3
Standard deviation	11.2	14.9	14.1	20.9	26.4	13.8

Predictive: Mean scores and standard deviations for pre-and posttreatment groups for 37 of 55 persons who completed a 55-day program for chronic back pain were as follows: pretreatment mean = 83.9, standard deviation = 13.3; posttreatment mean = 91.2, standard deviation = 18.4. Scores were higher for compliant than noncompliant patients.

Practicality: The Life Situation Survey is short and easy to administer.

References:

Chubon, R.A. Quality of life measurement of persons with back problems: Some preliminary findings. Journal of Applied Rehabilitation Counselling 16:31-34, 1985.

Chubon, R.A. Quality of life and persons with end-stage renal disease. Dialysis and Transplantation 15:450-452, 1986.

3. Review Form for Quality of Life Index

Name of Measure: Quality of Life Index (QLI)

Authors: Padilla, G.V., Presant, C., Grant, M.M., Metter, G., Lipsett, J., and Heide, F.

Primary Reference:

Quality of life index for patients with cancer. Research in Nursing and Health 6(3):117-126, 1983.

Purpose: This instrument is used to measure the quality of life of cancer patients.

Conceptual Framework: This instrument was derived from a measure originally proposed by Presant et al. (1981). It is based on a definition of quality of life that includes performance, personal attitudes or affective states, well-being, and support.

Description: The QLI contains 14 items organized into three groups: general physical condition, daily human activities, and personal attitudes. A self-administered format is used.

Reliability:

Stability: Two samples of chemotherapy patients, one sample of radiation therapy patients, and one sample of nonpatients were used to assess test-retest reliability. The time span between administrations of the first and second measure varied from 2 to 48 hours for the patients and several days for the nonpatients. For the patient samples, all items had statistically significant coefficients ($r \geq 0.60$, $p < 0.01$). For the nonpatients, the coefficients ranged from 0.11 to 0.90.

Internal consistency: Item analysis of the 14-item index across four samples yielded an alpha of 0.88.

Scalability: Ten-centimeter visual analogue scales are used. An overall score is obtained by summing the scores of the 14 items and dividing by 14. Subscale scores may also be calculated.

Validity:

Concurrent: Correlations between patient self-ratings, physician estimates of quality of life, and Karnofsky Index scores were in the low to moderate range for both the subscales and the total scores across the three groups of patients.

Construct: A principal component factor analysis provided three strong factors: psychological well-being, physical well-being, and symptom control, plus a fourth that relates to financial protection. Psychological well-being was the most important factor. The main factors correspond to the generally accepted definition of the components that comprise quality of life.

Discriminant: Discriminant validity was examined by comparing scores of the four groups using an analysis of variance. In terms of quality of life, a gradient was seen. Nonpatients demonstrated the highest scores, followed by chemotherapy outpatients, radiotherapy patients, and chemotherapy in patients.

Reference:

Presant, C.A., Klahr, C., and Hogan, L. Evaluating quality-of-life in oncology patients: Pilot observations. Oncology Nursing Forum 8(3):26-30, 1981.

4. Review Form for the Quality of Life Index for Colostomy Patients

Name of Measure: Quality of Life (QLI) for colostomy patients
Authors: Padilla, G.V., and Grant, M.M.

Primary Reference:

Quality of life as a cancer nursing outcome variable. Advances in Nursing Science 8(1):45-60, 1985.

Purpose: This instrument is used to assess the quality of life of colostomy patients.

Conceptual Framework: The QLI for patients with cancer (Padilla et al., 1983) was modified for use as a disease-specific instrument for patients who had undergone colostomy. A multidimensional operational definition of quality of life was employed.

Description: Ten items reflecting eating, pain, and sexual satisfaction, as well as interpersonal and body image aspects of self-worth were added to the original 14 items of the QLI. Descriptions of extreme subjective states were used to anchor the 23 visual analogue scales. The instrument is self-administered.

Reliability:

Internal consistency: Scores from 135 patients who had colostomies for a variety of conditions (mostly colorectal cancer) were used to assess internal consistency. The alpha coefficients were as follows: psychological well-being, alpha = 0.84; physical well-being, alpha = 0.87; body image, alpha = 0.80; response to surgery, alpha = 0.71; nutritional response, alpha = 0.48; and social concerns, alpha = 0.90.

Scalability: Scores from the 23 visual analogue scales were summed and divided by 23. Subscale scores can be calculated.

Validity:
Construct: Based on a factor analysis of the scores of 135 patients, six factors (listed under the section on internal consistency) were identified. To assess discriminant validity, mean scores of items common to both this instrument and the QLI were calculated. Again, nonpatients had the highest scores and the declining gradient was as expected, with cancer in patients scoring poorest. The colostomy patients had the second poorest scores.

Reference:

Padilla, G.V., Presant, C., Grant, M.M., Metter, G., Lipsett, J., Heide, F. Quality of life index for patients with cancer. Research in Nursing and Health 6(3):117-126, 1983.

5. Review Form for Quality of Life Index

Name of Measure: Quality of Life Index
Authors: Ferrans, C.E., and Powers, M.J.

Primary Reference:

Quality of Life Index: Development and psychometric properties. Advances in Nursing Science 8 (1):15-24, 1985.

Purpose: The Quality of Life Index (QLI) is used to assess the quality of life of both healthy subjects and dialysis patients.

Conceptual Framework: For this study, quality of life was defined as the satisfaction of needs. The domains of quality of life as presented in the literature and the individuals' evaluation of satisfaction with each domain, as well as its importance, were taken into account.

Description: The Quality of Life Index is comprised of two sections, one dealing with the satisfaction of needs and the other with the importance of the various domains. Each contains 32 items that assess health care, physical health and functioning, marriage, family, friends, stress, standard of living, occupation, education, leisure, future retirement, peace of mind, personal faith, life goals, personal appearance, self-acceptance, general happiness, and general satisfaction. For use with dialysis patients, there are also three items relating to treatment in each section.

Reliability:
Stability: Test-retest reliability within a two-week span for 69 graduate students was 0.87. For 20 dialysis patients, with a one-month time span between the two tests, reliability was 0.81.

Internal consistency: Analysis of graduate student scores gave an alpha coefficient of 0.93. An alpha coefficient of 0.90 was obtained in the patients' scores.

Scalability: Each item is accompanied by a six-point Likert scale ranging from "very satisfied" to "very dissatisfied" in the satisfaction section and from "very important" to "very unimportant" in the importance section. Scores are determined by adjusting satisfaction scores to incorporate importance. Specifically, satisfaction responses are recorded to make 0 the midpoint and then multiplied by importance responses. Thus, the highest scores are for the items that have high satisfaction and high importance; the lowest are for low satisfaction and high importance. Adjusted scores for each item are summed to create subscale and total scores.

Validity:
Content: Items were based on a literature review of the dimensions of quality of life as well as on patient reports of how dialysis affected the quality of their lives.

Concurrent: The scores on the Quality of Life Index were correlated against an overall satisfaction with life measure (Campbell, 1976). The correlation for graduate students was 0.75 and for dialysis patients, 0.65.

Reference:

Campbell, A., Converse, P.E., and Rodgers, W.L. The Quality of American Life: Perceptions, Evaluations and Satisfactions. New York, Russell Sage, 1976.

6. Review Form for Karnofsky Index of Performance Status (KPS)

Name of Measure: Karnofsky Index of Performance Status (KPS)
Authors: Karnofsky, D.A., and Burchemal, J.H.

Primary Reference:

The clinical evaluation of chemotherapeutic agents in cancer. In MacLeod, C.M., ed. Evaluation of Chemotherapeutic Agents in Cancer. New York, Columbia University Press, 191-205, 1949.

Purpose: The KPS is used to assess patients' overall ability to perform physical activities.

Conceptual Framework: Performance status is measured by patients' ability to carry out normal activities independently or with assistance. The presence of disease symptoms is also taken into account. Performance is equated with quality of life.

Description: The KPS is comprised of three general categories: self-care, general activities, and work. Within these categories, reflecting the level of care required, are 11 specific criteria.

Reliability:

Stability: Fifty patients were rated by a social worker in the clinic and again at home one week later. The two scores correlated significantly (Yates et al. 1980).

Interrater: Ratings by two independent physicians made the same day on emergency room patients and hemodialysis patients demonstrated problems in interrater agreement (Kappa = 50 percent and 29 percent, respectively) (Hutchinson et al. 1979).

Two ratings by nurses or social workers of cancer patients made within one week of each other correlated moderately (0.69) (Yates et al. 1980).

Independent ratings by two students of 30 patients with mixed diagnoses correlated highly (0.86). Information was obtained by chart reviews and patient interviews. Using 100 patients in a second study, the correlations were higher (0.96) (Grieco and Long 1984).

Sets of physicians or mental health professionals assessed 75 cancer patients. Pearson correlations were 0.89 and Kappa statistics were 59 percent (Schag et al. 1984).

Forty-seven interviewers rated 17 narratives of patients' performance. Interrater reliability using Cronbach's coefficient alpha and the intraclass correlation coefficient gave values greater than 0.97 (Mor et al. 1984).

Scaling: The rank ordered criteria are assigned scores from 100 down to 0 (100, 90, 80, etc.). After the most appropriate criteria are selected, the patient is assigned a score. The instrument is generally used by a health professional, but patients can also rate themselves.

Validity:

Content: The process of content development was not well described by the original author. Grieco and Long (1984) revised the KPS by providing more explicit descriptions of work, social interactions, and self-help skills. This new version correlated highly with the original.

Concurrent: Physician and self-assessment scores of functional capacity (as defined in the KPS) were compared. Kappa scores ranged from 11 percent to 17 percent (Hutchinson et al. 1979).

The KPS correlated highly (0.84) with the Quality of Well-Being Scale (Kaplan and Bush 1982) and moderately (0.68) with the self-report Health Perception Questionnaire (Ware 1976, Grieco and Long 1984).

Predictive: In general terms, KPS scores are predictive of survival. Low scores are better predictors of early death than are high scores of predicting longevity (Mor et al. 1984). KPS scores are useful for predicting survival (Yates et al. 1980).

Construct: When KPS scores were correlated against single variables relating to physical functioning, psychological status, and symptoms, Pearson correlations ranged from 0.09 to 0.63. All but two of ten variables produced significant correlations (Yates et al. 1980).

KPS scores discriminated among five groups of patients representing different levels of functioning (Grieco and Long 1984).

KPS scores by physicians were correlated with 18 variables assessing the type and severity of problems experienced by cancer patients. The correlations were significant but tended to be low (<0.51) (Schag et al. 1984).

KPS scores correlated significantly with other functional measures. No significant relations were found, however, between KPS scores and the presence of symptoms or the extent of disease (Mor et al. 1984).

Sensitivity: KPS scores reflect a progressive deterioration of the physical condition of cancer patients within five months (especially the last two months) of death (Yates et al. 1980).

Practicality: The KPS takes only a few minutes to complete.

References:

Grieco, A., and Long, C.J. Investigation of the Karnofsky Performance Status as a measure of quality of life. Health Psychology 3(2):129-142, 1984.

Hutchinson, T.A., Boyd, N.F., Feinstein, A.R., in collaboration with Gonda, A., Hollomby, D., and Rowat, B. Scientific problems in clinical scales, as demonstrated in the Karnofsky Index of Performance Status. Journal of Chronic Diseases 32(9-10):661-666, 1979.

Kaplan, R.M., and Bush, J. Health-related quality of life measurement for evaluation research and policy analysis. Health Psychology 1:61-80, 1982.

Mor, V., Laliberte, L., Morris, J.N., and Wiemann, M. The Karnofsky Performance Status Scale. An examination of its reliability and validity in a research setting. Cancer 53(9):2002-2007, 1984.

Schag, C.C., Heinrich, R.L., and Ganz, P.A. Karnofsky performance status revisited: Reliability, validity, and guidelines. Journal of Clinical Oncology 2(3):187-193, 1984.

Ware, J.E., Jr. Scales for measuring general health perceptions. Health Services Research 11 (14):396-415, 1976.

Yates, J.W., Chalmer, B., and McKegney, F.P. Evaluation of patients with advanced cancer using the Karnofsky performance status. Cancer 45(8):2220-2224, 1980.

7. Review for Functional Living Index—Cancer

Name of Measure: Functional Living Index—Cancer
Authors: Schipper, H., Clinch, J., McMurray, A., and Levitt, M.

Primary Reference:

Measuring the quality of life of cancer patients: The Functional Living Index—Cancer: Development and validation. Journal of Clinical Oncology 2(5):472-483, 1984.

Purpose: The Functional Living Index—Cancer (FLIC) is used to assess the overall functional outcomes of cancer patients. The FLIC serves as an adjunct to traditional measures of clinical assessment.

Conceptual Framework: The investigators designed the instrument to get a global measure of quality of life. It includes psychosocial considerations, such as nausea and vomiting, which are at the interface of medical outcomes and psychosocial factors, as well as other factors, such as freedom from pain, sociability, impact of illness, and satisfaction. It is cancer-specific, oriented to daily living, and designed for self-administra tion. The FLIC has 22 statements. Patients indicate how these statements apply to themselves on seven-point Likert scales.

Reliability:

Internal consistency: The investigators developed the instrument over four testings in Winnipeg and Edmonton, Canada, using 837 patients over a three-year period. Principal factor analysis with an orthogonal varimax rotation was used to reduce the items and define Physical Well-Being, an Ability Factor, and the Emotional State Factor.

Scalability: With seven-point scales for 22 items, the summary scores range from 22 to 154. Mean and standard deviations for summary and factor scores were not found.

Validity:

Content: A panel of 11 patients, relatives, physicians, nurses, and clergy generated a list of 250 items. The list was reduced to 92 items that were tested on 175 patients. Subsequent analysis of the questions reduced the number of statements to 20; in the last generation, items on nausea and recreational activity were added to bring the total to 22.

Concurrent: The scores were compared across four groups of patients in Winnipeg and Edmonton, Canada: follow-up, adjuvant treatment, active treatment, and hospitalized, and a group of patients in extended care in Winnipeg. The average scores decreased with extent of disease from a high of 116.6 to a low of 84.6. The overall analysis of variance was significant. A post hoc comparison of groups was not provided.

Construct: the total score, Factor 1 (physical well-being), and Factor 2 (psychologic scores) were correlated with the Katz Activities of Daily Living instrument, Goldberger's General Health Questionnaire with four subscales, the Beck Depression Inventory, Karnofsky Index, Speilberger State Treatment Anxiety Inventory, and Melzack Pain Inventory. All instruments were tested in Winnipeg and Edmonton, except for the Melzack Pain Inventory, which was tested only in Edmonton. Correlations were generally 0.50 or greater and in the predicted direction.

Sensitivity: The investigators did not report the instrument to be responsive to significant clinical change. Schipper et al. found the items to be free of socially desirable responses when analyzed with the Jackson Social Desirability Scale.

Practicality: The FLIC is presented on tear sheets that the patients can complete at home and return according to a predetermined schedule. Response rates are reportedly high.

References and Applications:

Finkelstein, D.M., Cassileth, B.R., Bonomi, P.D., Horton, J., Ezdinli, E.Z., Carbone, P.P., and Wolter, J.N. A pilot study of the Functional Living Index—Cancer (FLIC) Scale for the assessment of quality of life for metastatic lung cancer patients. American Journal of Clinical Oncology 2(6):630-633, 1988.

Fifty patients entered the study and four were later removed. Forty-three of the 46 patients administered the initial FLIC completed at least 90 percent of the questions. Thirty-four of the 41 (83 percent) patients alive after one month completed the FLIC, but the completion rate had dropped to 33 percent by six months. The investigators found that in addition to the reduction in response due to morbidity and mortality, compliance is itself correlated with quality of life. They suggest cross-sectional comparisons of mean scores at each cycle rather than studying changes in the FLIC over time. They also suggest analyzing changes in reverse time—that is, looking at the scores for the periods preceding death.

Ganz, P.A., Haskell, C.M., Figlin, R.A., La Soto, N., and Siau, J. Estimating the quality of life in a clinical trial of patients with metastatic lung cancer using the Karnofsky performance status and the Functional Living Index—Cancer. Cancer 61(4):849-856, 1988.

The investigators used the Karnofsky Performance Status and FLIC in a randomized trial of two programs for patients with advanced metastatic non-small cell lung cancer. Forty-eight of 63 eligible patients participated in the trial. The median survival was 16.9 weeks. A majority of patients had difficulty completing the FLIC; the investigators were unable to examine the effect of treatment on quality of life because of problems in the administration of the form.

8. Review Form for Selby et al.'s Quality of Life Measure

Name of Measure: Not named

Authors: Selby, P.J., Chapman, J.A., Etazadi-Amoli, J., Dalley, D., and Boyd, N.F.

Primary Reference:

The development of a method for assessing the quality of life of cancer patients. British Journal of Cancer 50(1):13-22, 1984.

Purpose: This instrument is to be used to assess the quality of life of patients with breast cancer.

Conceptual Framework: One section of the instrument is based on the Sickness Impact Profile (SIP), a global measure of health status developed by Bergner et al. (1981). The other section reflects clinical problems specific to the disease.

Description: The 12 categories of the SIP are each represented by one or more items for a total of 18 items. General areas included are work, home management, recreation, mobility, alertness, emotional behavior, eating, rest and sleep, social life, family relationships, body care and movement, and communication. Twelve items that reflect symptoms of the disease or of treatment are also included: pain, respiratory difficulty, sore mouth, nausea, vomiting, hair loss, attractiveness, appearance, dysuria, constipation, diarrhea, and fatigue. One item related to overall quality of life and one to satisfaction with life were also added, for a total of 32 items. The instrument can be self-administered or it can be scored by a physician.

Reliability:

Stability: Ninety-six patients completed the index on the morning of a clinic visit and again nine to twelve hours later. Generally, correlations were greater than 0.60, except for those dealing with nausea and vomiting. The investigators note that some patients received chemotherapy during the clinic visit.

Internal consistency: Using the scores from 96 breast cancer patients, investigators reported an alpha of 0.71.

Interrater: Self-assessments by 31 patients and ratings by physicians were correlated. Seventy-eight percent of the general items and 75 percent of the clinical items had a level of agreement greater than 0.60. In the study by Bell et al. (1985), all item scores by patients and their physicians correlated at least 0.5.

Scalability: Each item is accompanied by a 10-Centimeter visual analogue scale anchored at each end by descriptive phrases. In the analyses, each item is treated independently. Item scores are not summed.

Validity:

Content: Two groups of patients with breast cancer were interviewed using either an open-ended questionnaire or a structured questionnaire. The items were viewed as being both relevant and important.

Additionally, when the repeated scores of 96 breast cancer patients on chemotherapy were entered into a regression analysis using the item assessing the overall quality of life as the dependent variable and the other 31 items as the independent variables, between 68 percent and 83 percent of the variation in the global scale was explained. This information was seen as an indication of content validity.

Construct: Using quality-of-life data from 96 patients, factor analysis determined five factors that made clinical and biological sense for breast cancer.

When the items derived from the SIP categories were compared with the linear analogue scores of the SIP, they correlated significantly and in the expected direction. Group scores of patients with different levels of clinical severity differed significantly, demonstrating that the instrument could distinguish between groups of patients.

Sensitivity: The instrument registered the effects of chemotherapy when the treatment was started. Bell et al. (1985) reported that the measure was able to discriminate between high and low doses of chemotherapy. Data from an independent observer were more precise than data from the patients.

Practicality: Patients report the instrument to be quick, easy, and acceptable.

References and Applications:

Bell, D.R., Tannock, I.F., and Boyd, N.F. Quality of life measurement in breast cancer patients. British Journal of Cancer 51(4):577-580, 1985.
Twenty-five breast cancer patients participating in a randomized controlled trial of chemotherapy were assessed 3 weeks after chemotherapy started (just prior to the next dose) and 24 hours later. Scores were obtained from patients and physicians.
Bergner, M., Bobbit, R.A., Carter, W.B., and Gilson, B.S. The Sickness Impact Profile: Development and final revision of a health status measure. Medical Care 19(8):787-805, 1981.

9. Review Form for Linear Analogue Self-Assessment

Name of Measure: Linear Analogue Self-Assessment (LASA)

Authors: Baum, M., and Priestman, T.J.

Primary References:

Baum, M., Priestman, T.J., West, R.R., and Jones, E.M. A comparison of subjective responses in a trial comparing endocrine with cytotoxic treatment in the advanced carcinoma of the breast. European Journal of Clinical Oncology (Supplement) 1:223-226, 1980.

Priestman, T.J., and Baum, M. Evaluation of quality of life in patients receiving treatment for advanced breast cancer. Lancet 1(7965):899-900, 1976.

Purpose: The LASA is used to achieve a more complete picture of patients' subjective responses to treatment.

Conceptual Framework: The developers vary in the number of items that are used in the subjective ratings. For each variable, patients mark a 10-Centimeter line that is anchored at each end with words describing the extremes of that symptom. These include:

Symptoms and side effects: alopecia, anorexia, appetite, constipation, diarrhea, dyspnea, fatigue, nausea, pain, vomiting, and "other."

Anxiety and depression: apprehension, depression, insomnia, irritability, level of anxiety, mood, and well-being.

Personal relations: decisionmaking, getting along with partners and others, sexual relationships, and social relationships.

Physical performance: ability to perform daily activities, employment, level of activity, and social activities.

Reliability:

Stability: Twenty-nine breast cancer patients completed forms with 10 items. These forms were completed again 24 hours later at home. The correlation between sums of scores was 0.87.

Scalability: Scores are summed across items; means and standard deviations are reported. The LASA was designed for repeated testing (weekly) over the course of treatment.

Validity:

Concurrent: One hundred women with advanced breast cancer were randomly allocated to endocrine or combination cytotoxic therapy. Ninety-two were available for assessment; 51 completed the LASA. Fourteen of the 25 women in the endocrine group completed the LASA for six weeks.

Women in the cytotoxic group had higher symptom-related scores *and* higher quality-of-life scores than women in the endocrine group. Well-being differences reached significance after 11 weeks.

Predictive: Nonresponsive patients showed worse depression scores than women responding to treatment.

Sensitivity: Changes in weekly scores indicate that the LASA scores reflect clinical changes.

Practicality: Generally, patients were able to complete the LASA forms without difficulty. Naturally, for patients with advanced cancers, there were marked patient attrition rates caused by death or inability to respond.

References and Applications:

Coates, A., Dillenbeck, C.F., McNeil, D.R., Kaye, S.B., Sims, K., Fox, R.M., Woods, R.L., Milton, G.W., Solomon, J., and Tattersall, M.H. On the receiving end—II. Linear Analogue Self Assessment (LASA) in the evaluation of aspects of the quality of life of cancer patients receiving therapy. European Journal of Cancer and Clinical Oncology 19(11):1633-1637, 1983.

One hundred and ten patients (30 with melanoma, 41 with lung cancer, 39 with ovarian cancer) completed 506 LASA forms. The results were compared with performance status as measured by the Eastern Cooperative Oncology Group (ECOG) and response to therapy. LASA forms included items for global well-being (for example, well-being, mood, appetite) and disease-specific conditions (such as, pain, nausea, vomiting). Both ECOG scores and the LASA scores for general well-being showed parallel and marked deterioration during the period of radiotherapy with subsequent improvement.

Coates, A., Gebski, V., Bishop, J.F., Jeal, P.N., Woods, R.L., Snyder, R., Tattersall, M.H., Byrne, M., Harvey, V., and Gill, G., for the Australian-New Zealand Breast Cancer Trials Group, Clinical Oncology Society of Australia. Improving the quality of life during chemotherapy for advanced breast cancer. A comparison of intermittent and continuous treatment strategies. New England Journal of Medicine 317(24):1490-1495, 1987.

Gough, I.R., Furnival, C.M., Schilder, L., and Grove, W. Assessment of the quality of life of patients with advanced cancer. European Journal of Cancer and Clinical Oncology 19(8):1161-1165, 1983.

Lanham, R.J., and DiGiannantonio, A.F. Quality-of-life of cancer patients. Oncology 45(1):1-7, 1988.

A linear analogue scale consisting of 10 items, including feeling of well-being, mood, level of physical activity, pain, nausea, appetite, ability to perform work, social activities, level of anxiety, and whether treatment is helping, was administered to 98 cancer patients over 293 office visits and 137 family practice patients over 137 visits. The differences in mean scores, 6.09 for the cancer patients and 6.67 for the healthy patients, were statistically significant, but the investigators expected the differences to be larger. The group differences for men were statistically significant, but the differences for women were not. Male cancer patients had significantly lower scores than female cancer patients. The investigators identified work, physical activity, and socialization as special needs for men that should be addressed.

Raghavan, D., Grundy, R., and Lancaster, L. Assessment of quality of life in long-term survivors treated by first-line intravenous cisplatin for invasive bladder cancer. Progress in Clinical and Biological Research 260:625-631, 1988.

Questionnaires were sent to 29 patients by mail. In addition to the LASA, the investigators included multiple-choice questions on physical well-being, symptoms of the disease, side effects of treatment, functional status, sexual function, social interaction, satisfaction with treatment, and overall quality of life. Although the patients answered the multiple-choice questions readily, half of them were unable to use the LASA scales correctly. The highest nonresponse rate was on the LASA items related to sexual function.

10. Review Form for Breast Cancer Chemotherapy Questionnaire

Name of Measure: Breast Cancer Chemotherapy Questionnaire (BCQ)

Authors: Levine, M.N., Guyatt, G.H., Gent, M., De Pauw, S., Goodyear, M.D., Hryniuk, W.M., Arnold, A., Findlay, B., Skillings, J.R., Bramwell, V.H., et al.

Primary Reference:

Quality of life in stage II breast cancer: An instrument for clinical trials. Journal of Clinical Oncology 6(12):1798-1810, 1988.

Purpose: In planning their study, the investigators decided to develop a new questionnaire to measure the impact of adjuvant chemotherapy on physical, emotional, and social function of women with stage II breast cancer.

Conceptual Framework: The investigators reviewed the available measures of quality of life for cancer patients, but these did not focus on the specific problems of women with advanced breast cancer faced with receiving adjuvant therapy. Their goal was to develop a measure specific to the type of patient and the type of therapy. The items had to tap areas of physical, emotional, and social well-being that were important to the patient, quantifiable, valid, reproducible, responsive, simple, and convenient to use.

The items were generated through a literature review and discussions with medical oncologists, oncology nurses, and stage II breast cancer patients. The original 150 items were pared to 99, and 47 patients receiving adjuvant chemotherapy were asked to rate the importance of these items on five-point Likert scales. The investigators grouped the items into the areas of consequences of hair loss, emotional dysfunction, physical symptoms, trouble and inconvenience associated with treatment, fatigue, nausea, and positive well-being. They further decided that each area should have a minimum of four items. The final 30 items were selected, by area, in terms of the highest mean ratings of importance.

The women responded to items about how they had felt during the past two weeks on a seven-point scale.

Reliability:

Stability: At each visit, the women were asked if their condition had changed during the past two weeks. On the first occasion that no change was reported, the investigators compared the current and last scores on the quality-of-life measures. The mean change scores and standard deviations were deemed stable and reliable, but they were not statistically assessed.

Scalability: The responses for each item had a score from 1 to 7, and the scores were summed across the 30 items. This score was later transformed so that it ranged from 0 to 10.

Validity:

Content: The methods used for generating and selecting items assured the face and content validity of the items.

Construct: The first step was to average the scores for all visits for each patient. The mean BCQ scores were correlated with the average scores for patient and physician global ratings and the Karnofsky, RAND emotional, RAND physical, and Spitzer quality-of-life measures. The correlations ranged from 0.41 to 0.62. An analysis of change scores for a single two-week period showed that the global physical and emotional assessments by the patients were more strongly correlated with the quality-of-life ratings than the global assessments by the physicians.

Sensitivity: The women in the two treatment groups had the same therapy during the first 12 weeks, and the mean scores for women in the two groups were equivalent. For one group the treatment continued for 36 weeks and the other group stopped treatment after 12 weeks. The BCQ and Karnofsky scores were significantly lower for the short-term group than the 36 week group between weeks 12 and 36. The RAND and Spitzer scores did not vary significantly during this period. The scores converged again after 36 weeks, when all women were off therapy.

Practicality: The time, 30 minutes an interview, and costs of having the forms administered by a nurse/interviewer were considerable. The investigators have recommended that a self-administered version of the questionnaire be tested.

Application: In the trial, 418 women were assigned to either 12 weeks or 36 weeks of adjuvant therapy. A nurse/interviewer administered the BCQ, the RAND Physical Health and Mental Health Status questionnaires, and the Spitzer Quality of Life Index. The physician completed the Karnofsky Index. Global ratings of physical and emotional functioning were provided independently by the physician and the patients. The measures were completed at the beginning and the follow-up visits over a period of 80 weeks. The women stopped completing the measures when there was a recurrence of disease or they refused treatment. The patients averaged 10 visits and completed approximately 85 percent of the potential assessments.

REFERENCES

Anderson, J.P., Bush, J.W., and Berry, C.C. Internal consistency analysis: A method for studying the accuracy of function assessment for health outcome and quality of life evaluation. Journal of Clinical Epidemiology 41(2):127-137, 1988.

Andrews, F.M., and Witney, S.B. Social Indicators of Well-Being: American Perspectives of Life Quality. New York, Plenum, 1976.

Baum, M., Priestman, T.J., West, R.R., and Jones, E.M. A comparison of subjective responses in a trial comparing endocrine with cytotoxic treatment in the advanced carcinoma of the breast. European Journal of Clinical Oncology (Supplement) 1:223-226, 1980.

Bell, D.R., Tannock, I.F., and Boyd, N.F. Quality of life measurement in breast cancer patients. British Journal of Cancer 51(4):577-580, 1985.

Bergner, M., Bobbit, R.A., Carter, W.B., and Gilson, B.S. The Sickness Impact Profile: Development and final revision of a health status measure. Medical Care 19(8):787-805, 1981.

Bohrnstedt, G.W. Measurement. In Rossi, P.H., Wright, J.D., and Anderson, A.B., eds. Handbook of Survey Research. New York, Academic Press, 1981.

Campbell, A. The Sense of Well-Being in America: Recent Patterns and Trends. New York, McGraw-Hill, 1980.

Campbell, A., Converse, P.E., and Rodgers, W.L. The Quality of American Life: Perceptions, Evaluations and Satisfactions. New York, Russell Sage, 1976.

Chubon, R.A. Quality of life measurement of persons with back problems: Some preliminary findings. Journal of Applied Rehabilitation Counselling 16:31-34, 1985.

Chubon, R.A. Quality of life and persons with end-stage renal disease. Dialysis and Transplantation 15:450-452, 1986.

Chubon, R.A. A quality of life rating scale. Evaluation and the Health Professions 10:186-200, 1987.

Churchill, D.N., Torrance, G.W., Taylor, D.W., Barnes, C.C., Ludwin, D., Shimizu, A., and Smith, E.K. Measurement of quality of life in end-stage renal disease: The time trade-off approach. Clinical and Investigative Medicine 10(1):14-20, 1987.

Coates, A., Dillenbeck, C.F., McNeil, D.R., Kaye, S.B., Sims, K., Fox, R.M., Woods, R.L., Milton, G.W., Solomon, J., and Tattersall, M.H. On the receiving end--II. Linear Analogue Self Assessment (LASA) in the evaluation of aspects of the quality of life of cancer patients receiving therapy. European Journal of Cancer and Clinical Oncology 19(11):1633-1637, 1983.

Coates, A., Gebski, V., Bishop, J.F., Jeal, P.N., Woods, R.L., Snyder, R., Tattersall, M.H., Byrne, M., Harvey, V., and Gill, G., for the Australian-New Zealand Breast Cancer Trials Group, Clinical Oncology Society of Australia. Improving the quality of life during chemotherapy for advanced breast cancer. A comparison of intermittent and

continuous treatment strategies. New England Journal of Medicine 317(24):1490-1495, 1987.
Cronbach, L.J. Coefficient alpha and the internal structure of tests. Psychometrika 22:293-296, 1951.
Croog, S.H., Levine, S., Testa, M.A., Brown, B., Bulpitt, C.J., Jenkins, C.D., Klerman, G.L., and Williams, G.H. The effects of antihypertensive therapy on the quality of life. New England Journal of Medicine 314(26):1657-1664, 1986.
Drummond, M.F., Stoddart, G.L., and Torrance, G.W. Methods for the Economic Evaluation of Health Care Programmes. London, Oxford University Press, 1986.
Erickson, P., ed. Bibliography on Health Indexes, Clearinghouse on Health Indexes, National Center for Health Statistics, Hyattsville, Maryland.
Feinstein, A.R. Clinimetrics. New Haven, Yale University Press, 1987.
Ferrans, C.E., and Powers, M.J. Quality of Life Index: Development and psychometric properties. Advances in Nursing Science 8(1):15-24, 1985.
Finkelstein, D.M., Cassileth, B.R., Bonomi, P.D., Horton, J., Ezdinli, E.Z., Carbone, P.P., and Wolter, J.N. A pilot study of the Functional Living Index--Cancer (FLIC) Scale for the assessment of quality of life for metastatic lung cancer patients . American Journal of Clinical Oncology 2(6):630-633, 1988.
Fleiss, J.L. Statistical Methods for Rates and Proportions. 2nd ed. New York, John Wiley & Sons, 1981.
Fleiss, J.L. The Design and Analysis of Clinical Experiments. New York, John Wiley & Sons, 1986.
Fletcher, R.H., Fletcher, S.W., and Wagner, E.H. Clinical Epidemiology: The Essentials. 2nd ed. Baltimore, Williams and Wilkins, 1988.
Ganz, P.A., Haskell, C.M., Figlin, R.A., La Soto, N., and Siau, J. Estimating the quality of life in a clinical trial of patients with metastatic lung cancer using the Karnofsky performance status and the Functional Living Index--Cancer. Cancer 61(4):849-856, 1988.
Gough, I.R., Furnival, C.M., Schilder, L., and Grove, W. Assessment of the quality of life of patients with advanced cancer. European Journal of Cancer and Clinical Oncology 19(8):1161-1165, 1983.
Grieco, A., and Long, C.J. Investigation of the Karnofsky Performance Status as a measure of quality of life . Health Psychology 3(2):129-142, 1984.
Holloway, C.A. Decision Making Under Uncertainty: Models and Choices. Englewood Cliffs, New Jersey, Prentice-Hall, Inc., 1979.

Hutchinson, T.A., Boyd, N.F., Feinstein, A.R., in collaboration with Gonda, A., Hollomby, D., and Rowat, B. Scientific problems in clinical scales, as demonstrated in the Karnofsky Index of Performance Status. Journal of Chronic Diseases 32(9-10):661-666, 1979.

Kane, R.A., and Kane, R.L. Assessing the Elderly: A Practical Guide to Measurement. Lexington, Massachusetts, D.C. Heath and Company, 1981.

Kaplan, R.M., and Bush, J.W. Health-related quality of life measurement for evaluation research and policy analysis. Health Psychology 1:61-80, 1982.

Kaplan, R.M., Atkins, C.J., and Timms, R. Validity of a quality of well-being scale as an outcome measure in chronic obstructive pulmonary disease. Journal of Chronic Diseases 37 (2):85-95, 1984.

Karnofsky, D.A., and Burchemal, J.H. The clinical evaluation of chemotherapeutic agents in cancer. In MacLeod, C.M., ed. Evaluation of Chemotherapeutic Agents in Cancer. New York, Columbia University Press, 191-205, 1949.

Kerlinger, F.N. Foundations of Behavioral Research. 3rd ed. New York, Holt, Rinehart, and Winston, 1986.

Lanham, R.J., and DiGiannantonio, A.F. Quality-of-life of cancer patients. Oncology 45(1):1-7, 1988.

Last, J.M. ed. Dictionary of Epidemiology. 2nd ed. New York, Oxford University Press, 1988.

Levine, M.N., Guyatt, G.H., Gent, M., De Pauw, S., Goodyear, M.D., Hryniuk, W.M., Arnold, A., Findlay, B., Skillings, J.R., Bramwell, V.H., et al. Quality of life in stage II breast cancer: An instrument for clinical trials. Journal of Clinical Oncology 6(12):1798-1810, 1988.

McDowell, I., and Newell, C. Measuring Health: A Guide to Rating Scales and Questionnaires. New York, Oxford University Press, Inc., 1987.

Mor, V. Cancer patients quality of life over the disease course: Lessons from the real world. Journal of Chronic Diseases 40(6):535-544, 1987.

Mor, V., Laliberte, L., Morris, J.N., and Wiemann, M. The Karnofsky Performance Status Scale. An examination of its reliability and validity in a research setting. Cancer 53(9):2002-2007, 1984.

Morris, J.N., Suissa, S., Sherwood, S., Wright, S.M., and Greer, D. Last days: A study of the quality of life of terminally ill cancer patients. Journal of Chronic Diseases 39(1):47-62, 1986.

Nunnally, J.C. Psychometric Theory. 2nd ed. New York, McGraw-Hill, 1978.

Padilla, G.V., and Grant, M.M., Quality of life as a cancer nursing outcome variable. Advances in Nursing Science 8(1):45-60, 1985.

Padilla, G.V., Presant, C., Grant, M.M., Metter, G., Lipsett, J., and Heide, F. Quality of life index for patients with cancer. Research in Nursing and Health 6(3):117-126, 1983.

Presant, C.A., Klahr, C., and Hogan, L. Evaluating quality-of-life in oncology patients: Pilot observations. Oncology Nursing Forum 8(3):26-30, 1981.

Priestman, T.J., and Baum, M. Evaluation of quality of life in patients receiving treatment for advanced breast cancer. Lancet 1(7965):899-900, 1976.

Raghavan, D., Grundy, R., and Lancaster, L. Assessment of quality of life in long-term survivors treated by first-line intravenous cisplatin for invasive bladder cancer. Progress in Clinical and Biological Research 260:625-631, 1988.

Schag, C.C., Heinrich, R.L., and Ganz, P.A. Karnofsky performance status revisited: Reliability, validity, and guidelines. Journal of Clinical Oncology 2(3):187-193, 1984.

Schipper, H., Clinch, J., McMurray, A., and Levitt, M. Measuring the quality of life of cancer patients: The Functional Living Index--Cancer: Development and validation. Journal of Clinical Oncology 2(5):472-483, 1984.

Schuessler, K.F., and Fisher, G.A. Quality of life research and sociology. Annual Review of Sociology 11:129-149, 1985.

Selby, P.J., Chapman, J.A., Etazadi-Amoli, J., Dalley, D., and Boyd, N.F. The development of a method for assessing the quality of life of cancer patients. British Journal of Cancer 50 (1):13-22, 1984.

Smith, G.T., ed. Measuring Health: Practical Approach. New York, John Wiley & Sons, 1988.

Spitzer, W.O. State of science 1986: Quality of life and functional status as target variables for research. Journal of Chronic Diseases 40(6):465-471, 1987.

Spitzer, W.O., Dobson, A.J., Hall, J. Chesterman, E., Levi, J., Shepherd, R., Battista, R.N., and Catchlove, B.R. Measuring the quality of life of cancer patients. A concise QL-index for use by physicians. Journal of Chronic Diseases 34(12):585-597, 1981.

Torrance, G.W. Measurement of health state utilities for economic appraisal: A review. Journal of Health Economics 3:1-30, 1986.

Torrance, G.W. Utility approach to measuring health-related quality of life . Journal of Chronic Diseases 40(6):593-603, 1987.

Torrance, G.W., Thomas, W.H., and Sackett, D.L. A utility maximization model for the evaluation of health care programs. Health Services Research 7(2):118-133, 1972.

Torrance, G.W., Boyle, M.H., and Horwood, S.P. Application of multiattribute utility theory to measure social preferences for health states. Operations Research 30:1043-1069, 1982.

von Neumann, J., and Morgenstern, O. Theory of Games and Economic Behavior. 3rd ed. New York, John Wiley & Sons, 1953.

Ware, J.E., Jr. Standards for validating health measures: Definition and content. Journal of Chronic Diseases 40(6):473-480, 1987.

Ware, J.E., Jr. Scales for measuring general health perceptions. Health Services Research 11 (14):396-415, 1976.

Weinstein, M.C. Economic assessments of medical practices and technologies. Medical Decision Making 1:309-330, 1983.

Wenger, N.K., Mattson, M.E., Furberg, C.D., and Elinson, J., eds. Assessment of Quality of Life in Clinical Trials of Cardiovascular Therapies. New York, Le Jacq Publishing, Inc., 1984.

Yates, J.W., Chalmer, B., and McKegney, F.P. Evaluation of patients with advanced cancer using the Karnofsky performance status. Cancer 45(8):2220-2224, 1980.

Zeller, R.A., and Carmines, E.G. Measurement in the Social Sciences. London, Cambridge University Press, 1980.

7

Applications of Quality-of-Life Measures and Areas for Cooperative Research

Jennifer Falotico-Taylor and Frederick Mosteller

Several developments contribute to the emergence of the field of quality of life: the increased prevalence of chronic disease, the proliferation of health technologies, cost-containment concerns, and the current emphasis on social factors in health assessments.

Numerous quality-of-life instruments can evaluate health technologies in response to these concerns. Generic measures contain a minimum set of health concepts, usually measuring physical, psychological, social, and role functioning and general well-being. Specific measures target treatments, diseases, or populations.

Each measure has its own research advantages. For example, standardized, generic measures facilitate comparisons between various sick and well groups, younger and older age groups, and groups with different diseases; disease-specific measures are more sensitive to specific clinical interventions. Many researchers supplement accepted generic measures with specific measures that seem appropriate for a particular group, disease, or treatment.

Researchers emphasize the importance of focusing on these existing generic and specific measures and establishing more firmly their reliability and validity, rather than increasing the variety of measures. Clinicians

---

Acknowledgment: The issues and ideas presented in this chapter are drawn in large part from the summary statements of Frederick Mosteller, John E. Ware, Jr., and Sol Levine (Mosteller et al. 1989) presented at the Henry J. Kaiser Family Foundation Conference on Advances in Health Status Assessment, Menlo Park, California, July 13-15, 1988.

need these data for special populations such as handicapped groups, ethnic groups, the elderly, and well populations.

By being able to interpret these measures in a broader variety of populations, researchers can refine their work and strengthen their conclusions. The international community is already active in this area. Dr. Neil Aaronson of the Netherlands Cancer Institute has been investigating the applications of quality-of-life measurement in oncology clinical trials. He has also been working with the World Health Organization (WHO) Collaborating Center and is establishing a databank on the measurement of quality of life in clinical trials.

Researchers agree that for the quality-of-life field to continue to develop, it must be applied to daily clinical practice. Clinicians, in particular physicians, will carry most of the burden of using these measures. Clinicians are the key to the future of quality-of-life measurement in assessing health care because they form the front line. Researchers must clarify the relationship between clinical and general health measures as a way for clinicians to appraise and appreciate what quality-of-life scores or changes in scores mean in their clinical practice. By translating these quality-of-life scores into concrete gains or losses, the clinician can convert a score on a quality-of-life measure or a change in status to an indication for the next step in treatment or to greater insight about the health of a particular patient.

Short, easy to administer, and widely adaptable quality-of-life measures have the greatest chance of being used in a variety of clinical and practice routines. Researchers caution that although short-form measures may be more practical, they may not achieve the level of reliability and validity of lengthier forms. To convince others that undertaking the expense and time necessary to gather data on the various treatments and procedures is worthwhile, researchers need to demonstrate that use of these measures does improve the patients' outcomes.

Pharmaceutical companies have already funded some quality-of-life research as part of their product development; in the long term, quality-of-life concerns may become part of the marketing strategy for these firms. The interest these funding sources create in quality-of-life measures can increase their use by providing a reimbursement system that would encourage clinicians to administer these measures.

Several researchers have emphasized the importance of good methodological work. Toward this end, many investigators principally interested in measuring health outcomes have joined forces with researchers studying methodological issues. These cooperative, "piggybacked" studies capitalize on existing research opportunities by combining outcome and methodological research. Methodology investigators can provide technical assistance to those measuring health outcomes and may share costs if the additional methodological work is expensive. Sponsors of both types of research will receive more information and thus a greater return on their research investment.

Ultimately, quality-of-life research offers patients a greater voice and an opportunity to make more informed choices about their health care. For example, John Wennberg and his colleagues gave preoperative prostatectomy patients the chance to hear from others who had undergone this operation and who related, on film, their pre-and postoperative experiences. This approach gives the preoperative patient a better understanding of the consequences of this decision in quality-of-life terms. Clinicians also benefit because their patients have a more realistic view of what a specific treatment will and will not remedy. The joint effort of clinicians, health care researchers, administrators, and funding sources can strengthen technology assessments to improve the perceived as well as the physiological impact of interventions on patients.

REFERENCE

Mosteller, F., Ware, J.E., Jr., and Levine, S. Finale Panel: Comments on the conference on advances in health status assessment. Medical Care 27:S282-S294, March Supplement, 1989.

The Authors

Sydney H. Croog, Ph.D.
Professor of Behavioral Sciences and Community Health, University of Connecticut Health Center, 265 Farmington Avenue, Farmington, Connecticut 06032.

Jennifer Falotico-Taylor, A.L.B.
Research Assistant, Technology Assessment Group, Department of Health Policy and Management, Harvard School of Public Health, 677 Huntington Avenue, LL-7A, Boston, Massachusetts 02115.

Sol Levine, Ph.D.
Vice-President, The Henry J. Kaiser Family Foundation, Quadrus 2400 Sand Hill Road, Menlo Park, California 94025; and University Professor of Sociology and Public Health, University Professors Program, Boston University, Boston, Massachusetts 02215.

Kathleen N. Lohr, Ph.D.
Senior Professional Associate, Institute of Medicine, National Academy of Sciences, 2101 Constitution Avenue, N.W., Washington, D.C. 20418.

Bryan R. Luce, Ph.D.
Senior Research Scientist, Battelle Human Affairs Research Centers, 370 L'Enfant Promenade, S.W., Suite 900, Washington, D.C. 20024.

THE AUTHORS

Mark McClellan, B.A., B.S.
Kaiser Fellow in Health Policy and Management, Harvard-Massachusetts Institute of Technology, Division of Health Sciences and Technology, Center for Health Care Studies, E25-143, Massachusetts Institute of Technology, Cambridge, Massachusetts 02139.

Frederick Mosteller, Ph.D.
Director, Technology Assessment Group, Department of Health Policy and Management, Harvard School of Public Health, 677 Huntington Avenue, LL-7A, Boston, Massachusetts 02115.

Mark S. Roberts, M.D., M.P.P.
Clinical and Research Fellow, Division of General Medicine, New England Deaconess Hospital, Boston, Massachusetts, 02215; and Harvard Medical School, 110 Francis Street, Suite 7H, Boston, Massachusetts 02215.

Carol Underwood, M.A.
Research Associate, Battelle Human Affairs Research Centers, 370 L'Enfant Promenade, S.W., Suite 900, Washington, D.C. 20024.

Joan M. Weschler, B.S.N., M.A.
Research Associate, Battelle Human Affairs Research Centers, 370 L'Enfant Promenade, S.W., Suite 900, Washington, D.C. 20024.

J. Ivan Williams, Ph.D.
Professor, Department of Epidemiology and Biostatistics, McGill University, Montreal, Quebec H3G 1A4, Canada; currently with Clinical Epidemiology Unit, Sunnybrook Medical Center, 2075 Bayview Avenue, North York, Ontario M4N 3M5, Canada.

Sharon Wood-Dauphinee, Ph.D.
Associate Professor, School of Physical and Occupational Therapy, McGill University, Montreal, Quebec H3G 1A4, Canada.